SKIN DISEASES IN PREGNANCY

OrangeBooks Publication

Smriti Nagar, Bhilai, Chhattisgarh - 490020

Website:**www.orangebooks.in**

© **Copyright, 2023, Author**

All rights reserved. No part of this book may be reproduced, stored in a retrieval system, or transmitted, in any form by any means, electronic, mechanical, magnetic, optical, chemical, manual, photocopying, recording or otherwise, without the prior written consent of its writer.

First Edition, 03/01/2023

ISBN: 978-93-5621-294-7

SKIN DISEASES IN PREGNANCY
OVERVIEW AND MANAGEMENT
FIRST EDITION

Dr. Mubashar Mashqoor Mir
MBBS, MD DVL, DNB(Derm.), MNAMS.

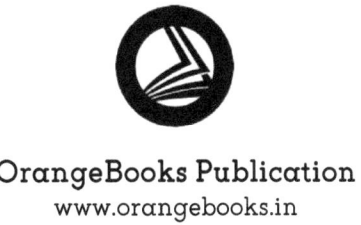

OrangeBooks Publication
www.orangebooks.in

Foreword

It gives me immense pleasure to pen down the foreword for the book titled '*Skin Diseases In Pregnancy - Overview & Management*' written and edited by Dr.Mubashar Mashqoor Mir.

Skin diseases in pregnancy have always been challenging to diagnose and difficult to treat due to the limitations of drugs that are approved for use in pregnancy.

I'm sure that this book will prove to be of great benefit for the students, academicians and private practitioners.

Dr. Mubashar Mashqoor Mir has done his Observership in Lasers n Hair transplant and Fellowship in Hair Restoration Surgery from Dermawave. He has always been a keen observer, great learner and a wonderful human being. I hope his painstaking efforts in writing this book pay off and benefit all .

I wish him good luck for his future Endeavors.

Dr. Sumit Sharma, MD
Founder & Director
Dermawave Skin Laser & Hair Transplant.

Preface

The first edition of this book 'Skin Diseases In Pregnancy - Overview and Management' has been brought with the intent of providing concise information to the readers regarding various skin changes that can present during the course of pregnancy. As we all know, pregnancy is a dynamic physiological state in which the mother undergoes various changes in almost all the organ systems including the skin and its appendages.

Whenever I used to read about skin changes in pregnancy, I always felt that the existing books either provided very little information or were too elaborate and full of complex jargon of words which was confusing for the routine reader including dermatologists and obstetricians. An effort has been made through this book to present the common changes; both physiological and pathological occurring during pregnancy in a crisp and to the point manner. This will make the book interesting and informative and worth the time of our readers. Since it is the first edition, I believe there may be a lot of things which could require improvement. As they say, in medical science everyday is a new learning. I hope that through this book I am able to bridge at least some of the lacunae that exists in the domain of obstetric dermatology as it exists today in our books. Wishing our readers an interesting and knowledgeable journey.

Sincerely,
Dr. Mubashar Mashqoor Mir.
MD, DNB, MNAMS.
Fellowship in Hair Restoration.
10-01-2023

Dedication

This book is dedicated to the loving memory of my father Dr. Mashqoor Ahmed, MD (Medicine). He was an astute clinician, a doctor by passion and my role model. He is perhaps the sole reason why I chose to be a doctor. I owe a great part of what I am to him. He is no longer with us but I know he would be a proud father today.

-Dr. Mubashar Mashqoor Mir

Acknowledgements

Book writing is a teamwork and it requires efforts from all fronts to make it a useful and successful presentation. There are a lot of acknowledgements to be made however I shall keep it short and sweet!

Foremost, I would like to extend my gratitude to my teachers who have taught me the knowledge and skills which I intend to share with my readers. The list is long however how I would take this opportunity to thank some of my mentors who had a significant impact in shaping me as a doctor and academician. My father was one of my first mentors who introduced me to the universe of medical science. He had a successful clinical practice and watching him attending to his patients was the preliminary stimulus which led me to tread on this difficult but exciting part. One wonderful teacher whom I met lately, Dr. Sumit Sharma, a well known dermatologist and hair transplant specialist gave a new dimension to my understanding of life, clinical practice and of course dermatology and hair transplant science. I have learnt both actively and passively a lot of things from him for which I shall always be grateful. My teachers from school and medical college also deserve my gratitude.

It is impossible to thank enough the people who support you day in and day out and stand by you so that you can excel in your field. My family has been a constant source of strength and support. I am fortunate enough to be able to do what I do and it is because of my parents, my brother Dr. Soheb and my sister Dr. Nazish.

I would also like to thank the bunch of friends that I have, especially Dr. Tahir and Dr. Kirti, for their help and support. My sincere thanks to Ajbir singh, my assistant for making my life easy.

-Dr Mubashar Mashqoor Mir.

Disclaimer

This work is subject to copyright. The author is safe to assume that the advice and information provided in this book is believed to be true to the best of their efforts and knowledge. The author does not give a warranty, expressed or implied, with respect to the material contained herein or for any errors or omissions that may have been made.

Contents

Part 1 Physiological Skin Changes In Pregnancy 1

Chapter 1
Pregnancy and the Skin: An Overview 3

Chapter 2
Dermato-Physiological Conditions In Pregnancy 8
Introduction 8
Pregnancy induced pigmentation 10
Connective tissue changes 13
    Striae gravidarum 13
    Skin tags 14
Changes in the hair during pregnancy 14
    Postpartum Telogen Effluvium 14
    Hirsutism 15
Changes in the nails during pregnancy 16
Neurovascular changes in pregnancy 16
    Pyogenic granuloma of pregnancy 16
    Gingival erythema and hyperemia 17
    Palmar erythema 17
    Spider angioma 18
    Venous varicosities 18
    Edema of pregnancy 19
    Carpal tunnel syndrome 20

Hematological and hemodynamic changes in pregnancy 20
Glandular changes in pregnancy 20
Conclusion 21

Part 2 Pregnancy Specific Dermatoses............................. 25

Chapter 3
An Overview of Pregnancy Specific Dermatoses 27

Chapter 4
Polymorphic Eruption Of Pregnancy (PEP) 31
Etiopathogenesis 31
Clinical presentation 32
Disease course and prognosis 33
Histopathology 34
Differential Diagnosis 34
Management.. 35

Chapter 5
Pemphigoid Gestationis (PG)... 38
Etiopathogenesis 38
Clinical presentation 39
Disease course and prognosis 39
Histopathology 40
Differential diagnosis 41
Management.. 41

Chapter 6
Atopic Eruption of Pregnancy (AEP) 44
Etiopathogenesis 44
Clinical presentation 45
Disease course and prognosis 45
Histopathology 46
Differential diagnosis 46
Management 47

Chapter 7
Intrahepatic Cholestasis of Pregnancy (ICP) 50
Etiopathogenesis 50
Clinical presentation 51
Disease course and prognosis 51
Histopathology 52
Differential diagnosis 52
Management 52

Part 3 Pregnancy Associated Dermatoses 57

Chapter 8
Inflammatory Dermatoses In Pregnancy 59
Atopic dermatitis 59
    Etiopathogenesis 59
    Clinical presentation 60
    Disease course and prognosis 60
    Management 60

Allergic contact dermatitis 62
Psoriasis 63
    Etiopathogenesis 63
    Effect of psoriasis on pregnancy 64
    Effect of pregnancy on psoriasis 64
    Management 64
Generalized Pustular psoriasis of Pregnancy (GPP) 66
    Etiopathogenesis 66
    Clinical presentation 67
    Differential diagnosis 68
    Histopathology 68
    Management 68
Urticaria 69
    Introduction 69
    Pregnancy and Urticaria 69
    Differential Diagnosis 70
    Management 70
Erythema nodosum (EN) 71
    Etiopathogenesis 71
    Clinical presentation 71
    Histopathology 72
    Management 72

Chapter 9
Autoimmune Connective Tissue Disorders In Pregnancy **76**

Lupus Erythematosus (LE) 76
    Introduction 76
    Disease course and prognosis 77
    Clinical presentation 78

Neonatal lupus erythematosus 79
Management 79
Antiphospholipid antibody syndrome (APLAS) 80
Systemic Sclerosis (SS) 81
Clinical presentation 81
Systemic Sclerosis and Pregnancy 82
Management 83
Dermatomyositis(DM) 84
Clinical Presentation 84
Dermatomyositis and pregnancy 85
Management 85

Chapter 10
Pemphigus In Pregnancy 90
Pemphigus Vulgaris (PV) 90
Etiopathogenesis 90
Clinical presentation 91
Differential diagnosis 91
Histopathology 91
Pemphigus and pregnancy 92
Pemphigus Foliaceus (PF) 93
Pemphigus foliaceus and pregnancy 93
Management of Pemphigus 94

Chapter 11
Skin Infections Associated With Pregnancy 97
Introduction 97
Vulvovaginal candidiasis 98
Bacterial vaginosis 99

Trichomonal vaginitis 100
Herpes zoster and chickenpox infection in pregnancy.............. 101
    1.Herpes zoster infection in pregnancy 101
    2.Varicella/Chickenpox in pregnancy 102
    3.Congenital varicella syndrome.. 103
    4.Infantile herpes zoster 103
    5.Chicken pox in a neonate 104
Genital warts in pregnancy 105
Herpes simplex infection in pregnancy...................................... 107
Pityriasis rosea in pregnancy 109
Human Immunodeficiency Virus (HIV) infection in pregnancy 110
Syphilis in pregnancy... 112
Scabies in pregnancy.. 113
Leprosy in pregnancy... 114

Chapter 12
Diseases Affecting The Sebaceous Glands
In Pregnancy... 119
Acne vulgaris in pregnancy 119
    Etiopathogenesis 120
    Clinical presentation... 120
    Differential diagnosis 121
    Management 121
Rosacea in pregnancy 123
    Etio pathogenesis 124
    Clinical features 124
    Management 125

Chapter 13
Diseases Of The Apocrine And Eccrine Glands In Pregnancy 129
Apocrine Gland Diseases in Pregnancy 129
   Hidradenitis suppurativa (HS) 129
   Fox Fordyce disease (FFD) 130
Eccrine Glands Diseases in Pregnancy 131
   Hyperhidrosis 131
   Miliaria 131

Chapter 14
Metabolic Diseases In Pregnancy 135
Porphyria cutanea tarda (PCT) 135
   Etiopathogenesis 136
   Clinical presentation 136
   Histopathology 138
   Diagnosis 138
   Treatment 139
Acrodermatitis Enteropathica (AE) 139
   Etiopathogenesis 140
   Clinical presentation 140
   Differential diagnosis 141
   Diagnosis 141
   Treatment 141

Chapter 15
Structural Connective Tissue Diseases In Pregnancy 143
Pseudoxanthoma elasticum (PXE) 144
   Etiopathogenesis 144

Clinical presentation 144
PXE and pregnancy 145
Anetoderma 146
Clinical features 147
Anetoderma and pregnancy 147
Ehler Danlos Syndrome (EDS) 148
Clinical presentation 148
Ehler Danlos Syndrome and pregnancy 148

Chapter 16
Uncommon Conditions Associated with Pregnancy 152
Autoimmune Progesterone Dermatitis In Pregnancy 152
Etiopathogenesis 152
Clinical presentation 153
Histopathology 154
Differential diagnosis 154
Treatment 155
Linear IgM dermatoses (LID) of pregnancy 155
Clinical presentation 155
Investigations 155
Diagnosis 156

Chapter 17
Neoplastic Conditions In Pregnancy 158
Non-Melanoma Skin Cancers (NMSCs) 158
Malignant Melanoma (MM) 159
Changes in melanocytic lesions in pregnancy 159
Malignant melanoma in pregnancy 159
Neurofibromatosis 161

Other tumorous growths in pregnancy 161

Chapter 18
Mucosal Changes In Pregnancy 167
Introduction 167
Changes in the Oral Mucosa 168
Physiological changes in oral mucosa 169
   Gingival hyperemia and edema 169
Pathological conditions of oral mucosa. 170
   1. Pyogenic Granuloma (PG) 170
   2. Aphthous Ulcers (AU) 171
   3. Bechet's disease (BD) 172
   4. Oral Involvement in Pemphigus Vulgaris (PV) 173
   5. Oral Involvement in Generalized Pustular psoriasis of Pregnancy (GPP) 174
   6. Oral Involvement in other Dermatoses 175
   7. Cheilitis during pregnancy 176
Changes In The Genital Mucosa During Pregnancy 176
   Pathological conditions affecting the vulva 177
   Vascular disorders of vulvar region 177
Infectious diseases affecting the genital mucosa in pregnancy .. 178
   1. Vulvovaginal Candidiasis (VVC) 178
   2. Bacterial vaginosis 180
   3. Trichomonal vaginitis 181
   4. Genital warts 182
   5. Genital herpes 184
   6. Molluscum contagiosum 187
Index 191

Part 1

Physiological Skin Changes In Pregnancy

Chapter 1

Pregnancy and the Skin: An Overview

Pregnancy is an altered physiological state which brings forth a multitude of physiological changes in the female body, including changes in the cutaneous and the subcutaneous tissue. These changes in the skin are a consequence of the alterations in the endocrine, metabolic and immunological system during the period of pregnancy.

The cutaneous manifestations of pregnancy are a result of the increased production of various proteins and steroid hormones secreted by the feto-placental unit and also by the pituitary, thyroid, ovaries and adrenal glands of the mother. A new endocrine organ which is present in the gravid female is the placenta, which produces an additional quota of hormones including progesterone. Another hormone namely dehydroepiandrosterone is produced by the adrenal glands of the fetus from pregnenolone and this is further aromatized to estriol. The production of these hormones increases multifold as the pregnancy progresses. At term of gestation, the level of progesterone is 7 times, prolactin level is 19 times and estradiol level is 130 times of that seen during 8 weeks of gestation.

Alterations in the immunological profile of the mother also take place during the period of pregnancy. This includes an over dominance of Th2 expression due to the increased levels of progesterone seen during pregnancy. Th2 cytokines like IL4, IL5 and IL10 are produced which have an inhibitory effect on the Th1 pathway mediators like TNF alpha production. Hormones like estrogen also suppress interleukin 2 production. During the postpartum period, as a result of the withdrawal of these hormones, there is a consequent elevation of the Th1 cytokines which may lead to reversal of the physiological changes seen in pregnancy. Sometimes diseases like psoriasis, which may undergo remission, can flare up again during the postpartum period as a result of withdrawal of high levels of pregnancy induced hormones. Due to the heightened demand of the body and the biochemical changes taking place in the body, various systemic changes also take place, including in the cardiovascular system and renal system. Changes in the cutaneous appendages like hair and nails are also seen. One or the other form of cutaneous changes occur in almost 90% of the gravid females. This can vary from the commonly seen changes like striae gravidarum to less commonly seen changes like carpal tunnel syndrome. The cutaneous manifestations can range from mild to severe. Some changes are seen exclusively in pregnancy, while others can be precipitated or modified due to pregnancy.

Cutaneous changes in pregnancy can broadly be classified into physiological changes associated with pregnancy, pregnancy specific dermatoses and pregnancy associated dermatoses. All these conditions shall be dealt separately in the subsequent chapters of this book.

Figure 1.

SKIN DISEASES IN PREGNANCY

- Physiological Changes in Pregnancy
- Pregnancy Specific Dermatoses
- Pregnancy Associated Dermatoses

As far as the treatment is concerned, pregnancy dermatoses can often be challenging for the treating doctor. Due to the fear of side effects to the fetus and mother, the patients as well as the physicians tend to stay on the side of restraint, resulting in under treatment of these disorders. Sometimes unnecessary or over treatment can also happen because the physiological changes in pregnancy may be wrongly perceived as pathological.

Another major challenge in treatment of skin diseases during pregnancy remains the lack of data available on the safety profile of various medications, because safety studies of most of these medications exclude pregnant and lactating females as a convention. Whatever data is available, exists in the form of incidental exposure, personal opinions of the doctors and some case reports. There is paucity of proper randomized control studies on pregnant females as far as the majority of drugs are concerned.

Having adequate knowledge of medication safety during pregnancy, physiological changes in pregnancy and pregnancy dermatoses is vital for every dermatologist and obstetrician dealing with pregnant females. Only a treating doctor who has adequate knowledge of obstetric dermatology can confidently deal with dermatological disorders in pregnant patients and avoid unnecessary side effects to the mother and child. Through the medium of this book an effort would be made to apprise the readers about various physiological changes in pregnancy, disease states in pregnancy as well as rational approach of treatment and diagnosis in these cases.

References

1. Griffith, C. E.M., & Baker, J. (Eds.). (2016). Rook's Textbook of Dermatology (9th ed. Vol. 3).Willey Blackwell.

2. Ingber, A. (2008). Obstetric Dermatology: A Practical Guide. Springer.

3. Tyler, K. H. (Ed.). (2020). Cutaneous Disorders of Pregnancy. Springer International Publishing.

4. Vora, R. V., Gupta, R., Mehta, M. J., Chaudhari, A. H., Pilani, A. P., & Patel, N. (2014). Pregnancy and skin. Journal of family medicine and primary care, 3(4), 318–324. https://doi.org/10.4103/2249-4863.148099

5. Kar S, Krishnan A, Shivkumar PV. Pregnancy and skin. J Obstet Gynaecol India. 2012 Jun;62(3):268-75. doi: 10.1007/s13224-012-0179-z. Epub 2012 Aug 28. PMID: 23730028; PMCID: PMC3444563.

6. Shivakumar V, Madhavamurthy P. Skin in pregnancy. Indian J Dermatol Venereol Leprol 1999;65:23-25

7. Oumeish OY, Parish JL. Pregnancy and the skin. ClinDermatol. 2006;24: 78-79.

8. Mehta N, Chen KK, Kroumpouzos G. Skin disease in pregnancy: the approach of the obstetric medicine physician. Clin Dermatol. 2016;34: 320-326.

9. Kepley JM, Mohiuddin SS. Physiology, maternal changes. Treasure Island: StatPearls; 2019;

10. Soutou B, Aractingi S. Skin disease in pregnancy. Best Pract Res Clin Obstet Gynaecol. 2015;29(5):732–40.

Chapter 2

Dermato-Physiological Conditions In Pregnancy

Introduction

The state of pregnancy is associated with a myriad of physiological changes that have a direct impact on the cutaneous structures and its appendages. The hormonal, immunological and metabolic alterations that happen during pregnancy have a direct impact on the physiology of skin. These alterations exert a variety of effects on the skin including cutaneous pigmentation, changes in the cutaneous vasculature and changes on the skin appendages like the nails and hair. More often than not, effects of pregnancy on skin and its appendages are a common manifestation during the early course of pregnancy.

Such changes occurring during the pregnancy often lead to distress among the patients. Hence, it is very important for the treating doctor to recognise these changes timely and counsel the patients about the benign nature of physiological changes to alleviate their stress. More importantly, the doctor should be able to differentiate physiological changes from pathological conditions in pregnancy and advise necessary intervention in case of cutaneous diseases associated with pregnancy.

Pathological changes or disease states of the skin during pregnancy, also known as the pregnancy dermatoses, should be differentiated from the physiological changes which are nothing but deviation from the normal physiological state as a result of pregnancy.

In this chapter we will discuss some commonly seen physiological changes occurring during pregnancy and how to differentiate them from the pathological pregnancy dermatoses.

Figure 2.

PHYSIOLOGICAL CHANGES IN PREGNANCY

- Pigmentary Changes
    - Linea Nigra
    - Diffuse Hyperpigmentation of Axilla, Groins and Areola
    - Melasma
    - Changes in Freckles, Lentigines and Nevi
    - Pigmentary Demarcation Lines
- Connective tissue changes
    - Striae Gravidarum
    - Skin Tags
- Hair changes
    - Postpartum Telogen Effluvium
    - Male Pattern Hair Loss
    - Hirsutism

- Nail changes
    - Brittle Nails
    - Nail Splitting
    - Onycholysis
    - Subungual Hyperkeratosis
    - Beau's Lines
    - Longitudinal Melanonychia
    - Leukonychia
    - Ingrowing Nail

- Neurovascular changes
    - Pyogenic Granuloma
    - Gingival Hyperemia
    - Palmar Erythema
    - Spider Angioma
    - Venous Varicosities
    - Edema of Pregnancy
    - Carpal tunnel Syndrome

- Hematological and Hemodynamic changes

- Changes in glandular function

Pregnancy induced pigmentation

Pregnancy induced pigmentation is one of the most frequently seen physiological changes in pregnancy. It is seen to occur in around 90% of the cases and is usually more commonly seen in women of color which explains its more common occurrence in the Indian pregnant females. The exact cause of this hyperpigmentation is so far unclear, however stimulation of the melanocytes stimulating hormone (MSH) as a result of elevated blood hormones; i.e. estrogen and progesterone are thought to have an impact on the hyperpigmentation seen in pregnancy. Hyper pigmentation is seen to develop more during the second half of pregnancy and is often limited to specific areas and specific patterns. Linea Alba which is the longitudinal line extending from the xiphoid process to the pubic symphysis darkens to become **linea nigra** during pregnancy. The pigmentation of linea nigra often resolves to some extent after delivery. This is often accompanied by accentuation of the **diffuse pigmentation** in regions where the skin is normally more pigmented. This includes areas like the axillae, groins, perineum and the peri-anal area. During the course of pregnancy there is accentuated darkening of the areolar skin as well which is known as the **secondary areola**. **Pigmentary demarcation lines** can also become more apparent during pregnancy. Pre-existing pigmented skin lesions like **nevi, freckles and lentigines** may show accentuated pigmentation and may resemble a mole which has shown a sudden change in its color. In case suspicion of dysplastic change in a mole arises during pregnancy; biopsy to rule out such change can be done

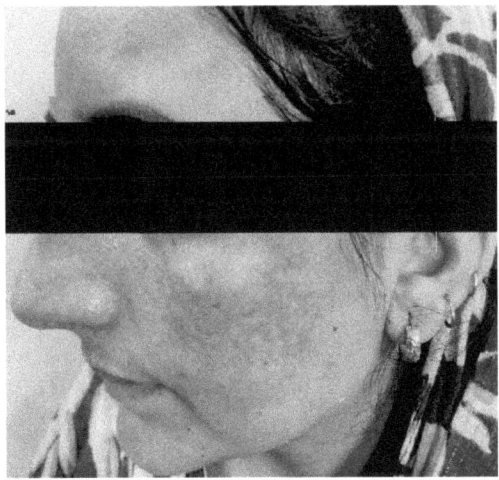

Figure 3 Image of a patient having melasma in pregnancy

Another common finding in pregnancy is the facial hyperpigmentation which is called **melasma** (chloasma). It is seen to occur in around 70% of pregnant females. It presents as a poorly demarcated bilaterally symmetrical hyperpigmentation involving the face, sometimes the neck and the forearm. Hypermelanosis on the face commonly involves the bridge of the nose and cheeks, upper lip, forehead and the mandibular region. Besides pregnancy the other causes which trigger melasma include photo exposure and the use of oral contraceptive pills. Genetic predisposition is also found to be responsible in around 20% of the cases. Melasma is seen to increase or develop de novo more during the second trimester of pregnancy. The deposition of pigment can be epidermal, dermal or in a mixed pattern. Post pregnancy, melasma is seen to settle down at least partially in most of the females. Patients with melasma should be advised to avoid use of oral contraceptive pills postpartum and use some other method of contraception as OCPs may exaggerate melasma.

Management includes regular use of good sunscreen and if melasma persists after delivery, topical agents in the form of hydroquinone, azelaic acid, vitamin C, kojic acid etc can be used. As far as the use of these topical agents during pregnancy is concerned, most of the practitioners prefer avoiding these agents due to the lack of safety data in pregnancy. However, topical agents like kojic acid and hydroquinone are minimally absorbed and hence are considered safe during lactation. An even safer choice to consider for topical treatment of melasma can be azelaic acid which is a pregnancy category B drug.

Connective tissue changes

The cutaneous changes which occur during pregnancy also include the changes occurring in the connective tissue.

Striae gravidarum

A common finding involving the connective tissue during pregnancy is striae gravidarum also known as stretch marks. It is a common finding in the majority of females during pregnancy. Stretch marks are seen to appear more during the second and third trimester of pregnancy and predominantly involve the abdomen, breasts, buttocks, thighs and hips. In the beginning the stretch marks appear slightly erythematous or violaceous in color and later become whitish or pale with presence of variable atrophy. The lesions can sometimes be associated with pruritus. The predisposition of abdomen and pelvic region is attributed to the sudden increase in girth of these areas as a result of weight gain in pregnancy which causes excessive stretching of the skin and consequently there is destruction of the dermal connective tissue which consists of collagen and elastic fibers. Other factors which contribute to the occurrence of stretch marks include a genetic susceptibility, excessive weight gain during pregnancy, conception at a young age and use of steroids during the period of pregnancy. Striae gravidarum is often a cosmetic concern for most pregnant females.

Both preventive and therapeutic topical treatments have been tried with variable success. Preventive measures include the application of oils like coconut oil, almond oil, olive oil, vitamin E cream and topical plant based extracts like *centella asiatica* extract. Topical tretinoin is found to be effective during the early erythematous stage of striae however tretinoin is a pregnancy category C drug and is to be avoided during the period of pregnancy. Once the period of pregnancy and lactation is over, therapeutic treatments are often tried which include use of topical tretinoin cream, PRP therapy, use of fractional lasers, IPL and pulsed dye lasers which have yielded good results.

Skin tags

Skin tags also known as *mollusca fibrosa* or *acrochordons* may also develop during the second and third trimester of pregnancy. They appear as skin coloured or pigmented fleshy pedunculated papules with predisposition towards involvement of body folds including neck, axilla, groins and the infra mammary area. Some of these lesions can regress after delivery and in case they persist or are symptomatic, they can be excised under local anesthesia.

Changes in the hair during pregnancy

Postpartum Telogen Effluvium

Sudden increase in the shedding of hair is a common complaint communicated to the doctor by the female during the postpartum period. This results due to a prolonged growth phase (anagen) of the hair cycle seen during pregnancy. Once the pregnancy is over, more numbers of hair are seen to enter the resting phase also known as the telogen phase. This results in an usually high shedding of hair two to four months after delivery. This is often very distressing for the female patient however the prognosis of **postpartum telogen effluvium** is good in most of the cases and hair loss often subsides within a year after delivery. Most of the patients present with diffuse hair loss involving the whole of the scalp, however **fronto-parietal recession** can also be seen in a minority of the patients.

The condition is often transient whereby pregnancy acts as a trigger and once the pregnancy is over the condition often reverses within a year. Thus, no active treatment is required. However hypothyroidism and iron deficiency anemia should be excluded before labeling the patient as a case of postpartum effluvium. Uncommonly, some cases may continue with prolonged hair loss extending beyond 1 to 2 years and rarely the diffuse hair loss seen after delivery may not be completely reversible. In such cases an active search should be done to rule out any other associated factor or an underlying disease state along with empirical treatment in the form of topical minoxidil and oral supplements should be instituted.

Hirsutism

It is defined as the excessive, abnormal growth of terminal dark hair occurring in females in a male pattern distribution. It can be seen commonly during pregnancy and often affects the areas of masculine hair growth that is the face, chest, back and the limbs. It is believed to result due to an increase in the level of androgenic hormones secreted by the placental tissue as well as the maternal ovary. It is more common in females of darker color hence Indian females are more commonly affected than the caucasians. Hirsutism in pregnancy often begins early and reverses within the first year after delivery. If unwanted hair growth persists for more than 6 months after pregnancy and the patient wants cosmetic improvement; laser hair reduction can be done. Severe growth in male pattern distribution should alert the physician to actively conduct an endocrine assessment to rule out an underlying androgenic abnormality or tumor.

Changes in the nails during pregnancy

Nail changes are not very common in pregnancy; however when they occur they usually appear early during the first trimester in the form of **softening and increased fragility of the nail plate**, separation of the nail plate from the nail bed (**onycholysis**) and accumulation of keratin debris under the nail plate (**subungual hyperkeratosis**). Other findings include **longitudinal melanonychia, leukonychia, ingrowing nail and nail splitting**. Sometimes, transverse grooves can be seen on the nail plate which signifies periods of temporary arrest in the nail plate growth due to the effect of pregnancy acting as a stresser; these are known as **beau's lines**. These nail changes are often temporary and reverse within the first year after delivery. Overall the **nail growth** is seen to increase during the pregnancy and slow down after delivery.

Because of the temporary nature of these changes, no active intervention is usually required. However, other possible causes of nail abnormality like onychomycosis, psoriasis and lichen planus should be ruled out.

Neurovascular changes in pregnancy

Pyogenic granuloma of pregnancy

It is a benign proliferative lesion involving the capillaries during pregnancy. It appears as a bright red papule or nodule involving the skin or mucosal sites, most commonly the gingiva or lip during pregnancy. The lesion is friable and can easily bleed on manipulation. The cutaneous lesion is often pedunculated with a collar of epithelial tissue at the base of its stalk. The skin lesion can regress after delivery and may not need any active intervention. However, in case of persistence or recurrent infection or bleeding from the lesion; surgical treatment may be undertaken during pregnancy. It includes electro-surgical ablation or cryotherapy or excision.

Gingival erythema and hyperemia

Hormone mediated increase in the vasculature of gingival mucosa presents in the form of gingival erythema and hyperemia which can be associated with **gingivitis and gingival bleeding**. Whether gingival bleeding is associated with Vitamin C deficiency or is a direct consequence of gingival hyperemia, is unknown. Some pregnant patients may also complain of **periodontitis.**

Palmar erythema

Palmar erythema is a common finding seen in pregnancy; often in the beginning of pregnancy. It is more common in caucasians than in women of color. It presents in the form of diffuse redness as well as mottled erythema of the thenar and hypothenar eminences of both palms as well as fingertips. Some females also complain of a mild burning sensation associated with these lesions. The condition is usually completely reversible and fades within 2 weeks after delivery. In case of persistence; conditions like cirrhosis of the liver and lupus erythematosus should be ruled out.

Spider angioma

It is seen as a flat or mildly elevated lesion with a central red punctum and radiating telangiectatic capillaries; usually during the second trimester of pregnancy. They are more commonly seen in the area of head and neck and the upper limb. They usually persist until the time of delivery and fade rapidly within the first three months after delivery. In case they are seen to persist for a longer period, surgical treatment in the form of electrocoagulation of the central arteriole using a fine tip or needle probe can be done. Other methods include the use of vascular lasers including IPL laser and pulsed dye laser.

Both palmar erythema and spider angioma in pregnancy are believed to occur because of high levels of circulating estrogen.

Venous varicosities

Due to the hemodynamic changes that occur during pregnancy like increase in the plasma volume, hyperdynamic circulation and decreased peripheral resistance; there is an increase in the venous blood pressure. Hormonal contribution in the form of increased water retention caused due to elevation of estrogen and progesterone hormone as well as vascular relaxation caused by the effect of relaxin hormone; contributes towards the increased pressure in capacitance vessels. This manifests clinically in the form of varicosities seen during pregnancy involving the lower legs, perivulvar, perianal region, periumbilical region etc. Venous varicosities appear to be most prominent and symptomatic during the third trimester of pregnancy, delivery and the immediate postpartum period. It can also manifest in the form of hemorrhoidal bleeding and pain which can be treated conservatively by increasing water and dietary fiber intake, sitz bath, topical anesthetic creams and treatment of associated constipation. Venous varicosities involving the vaginal region present in the form of bluish hue of the vaginal mucosa and is called **chadwick sign**. Another similar finding in the form of bluish discoloration of the cervix is known as **goodell sign**. These are a direct result of the increased vascularity of the vaginal and cervix mucosa.

Edema of pregnancy

Due to the increased water and salt retention seen in pregnancy as well as the increased capillary perfusion; there occurs non pitting edema involving the extremities and the face. It is seen more on the dependent parts of the body including the lower limbs and ankles. It is seen in more than 50% of pregnant females. Simple measures including adequate bed rest, foot end elevation can decrease the dependent edema. The patient can be instructed to immerse her feet in saline water or massage the limbs and sleep in the left lateral position to reduce obstruction of inferior vena cava flow which can prove helpful. Avoidance of excessive salt intake and use of elastic compression stockings can also help in the management of pregnancy induced edema. In case of prolonged edema of the face and extremities associated with hypertension and frothy urine conditions like preeclampsia, should be ruled out.

Carpal tunnel syndrome

Carpal tunnel syndrome is a form of compression neuropathy of the median nerve as it passes under the flexor retinaculum at the level of the wrist. The compression occurs due to soft tissue edema as a result of hormone induced tissue swelling, associated with pregnancy. The patient presents with symptoms in the form of pain, numbness and swelling of the affected hand. The condition is often transient and usually resolves after delivery.

Other uncommon vascular findings in pregnancy include **hemangiomas, cutis marmorata, purpura** and **petechiae**.

Hematological and hemodynamic changes in pregnancy

Pregnancy is a state of physiological haemodilution. This results in **hyper dynamic circulation** and **high cardiac output** due to increased salt and water retention caused by high estrogen and progesterone levels during pregnancy. Hematological changes in pregnancy include transient **thrombocytopenia** and a **hypercoagulable state**. There is an increase in coagulation factors such as factor 7, 8, 9 and 10 during pregnancy.

Glandular changes in pregnancy

The state of pregnancy exerts its effects on eccrine glands, apocrine glands and sebaceous glands. Increased function of sweat glands in pregnancy may lead to **increased sweating, miliaria** and **dyshidrosis**. Increased activity of sweat glands is seen more during the last trimester of pregnancy however ironically the palms are usually less affected.

Some authors believe that apocrine gland activity is reduced during pregnancy. Consequently an **improvement in fox fordyce's disease and hidradenitis suppurativa** can be seen during pregnancy and these conditions may again flare up after delivery.

High estrogen levels during pregnancy may activate sebaceous glands and increase the sebaceous gland secretions. Whether increased sebaceous gland activity has an effect on the occurrence of acne in pregnancy is debatable. Sebaceous gland hyperplasia in the form of **Montgomery tubercles** is seen during the 6th week of pregnancy and is considered to be an early sign of pregnancy. They appear as brown and round papules in the areola and serve to provide lubrication for the nipples during breastfeeding.

Conclusion

Clinicians need to be well aware of the physiological alterations caused due to pregnancy on the skin and its appendages. These changes have an effect on skin pigmentation, connective tissue, dermal neurovasculature and cutaneous appendages like hair and nails. These changes are mainly a result of the altered metabolic, immunological and hormonal profile during pregnancy. Physiological changes in pregnancy involving the skin should be well differentiated from pregnancy dermatoses so that the mother and the fetus are not exposed to unnecessary medications and interventions as most of these conditions are benign and reverse after the completion of pregnancy.

References

1. Griffith, C. E.M., & Baker, J. (Eds.). (2016). Rook's Textbook of Dermatology (9th ed., Vol. 3). Willey Blackwell.

2. Ingber, A. (2008). Obstetric Dermatology: A Practical Guide. Springer.

3. Tyler, K. H. (Ed.). (2020). Cutaneous Disorders of Pregnancy. Springer International Publishing.

4. Vaughan Jones SA. Physiologic skin changes of pregnancy. In:Black MM, Ambros-Rudolph CM, Edwards L, Lynch P, Eds. Obstetric and Gynaecologic Dermatology , 3rd edn. New York : Mosby, 2008 : 23 – 30.

5. Vora, R. V., Gupta, R., Mehta, M. J., Chaudhari, A. H., Pilani, A. P., & Patel, N. (2014). Pregnancy and skin. Journal of family medicine and primary care, 3(4), 318–324. https://doi.org/10.4103/2249-4863.148099

6. Kar S, Krishnan A, Shivkumar PV. Pregnancy and skin. J Obstet Gynaecol India. 2012 Jun;62(3):268-75. doi: 10.1007/s13224-012-0179-z. Epub 2012 Aug 28. PMID: 23730028; PMCID: PMC3444563.

7. Rathore SP, Gupta S, Gupta V. Pattern and prevalence of physiological cutaneous changes in pregnancy: A study of 2000 antenatal women. Indian J Dermatol Venereol Leprol 2011;77:402

8. Kumari R, Jaisankar T J, Thappa DM. A clinical study of skin changes in pregnancy. Indian J Dermatol Venereol Leprol 2007;73:141

9. Motosko, C. C., Bieber, A. K., Pomeranz, M. K., Stein, J. A., & Martires, K. J. (2017). Physiologic changes of pregnancy: A review of the literature. International journal of women's dermatology, 3(4), 219–224.

https://doi.org/10.1016/j.ijwd.2017.09.003

10. Geraghty LN, Pomeranz MK. Physiologic changes and dermatoses of pregnancy. Int J Dermatol. 2011;50(7):771–82.

11. Rubin A, Van Laborde S, Stiller MJ. Acquired dermal melanocytosis: appearance during pregnancy. J Am Acad Dermatol 2001;45: 609- 13.

12. Barankin B, Silver SG, Carruthers A (2002) The skin in pregnancy. J Cutan Med Surg 6:236–240

13. Elling SV, Powell FC (1997) Physiological changes in the skin during pregnancy. Clin Dermatol 15:35–43

14. Errickson CV, Matus NR (1994) Skin disorders of pregnancy. Am Fam Physician 49:605–61038. Wade TR, Wade SL, Jones HE (1978) Skin changes and diseases associated with pregnancy. Obstet Gynecol 52:233–242

15. Tunzi M, Gray GR (2007) Common skin conditions during pregnancy. Am Fam Physician 75:211–218

Part 2

Pregnancy Specific Dermatoses

Chapter 3

An Overview of Pregnancy Specific Dermatoses

Pregnancy specific dermatoses are described as cutaneous conditions which arise specifically during the period of pregnancy or postpartum period and are not usually seen in non pregnant females. Rudolph et al. in the year 2006 classified pregnancy specific dermatoses. Some authors also include generalized pustular psoriasis of pregnancy (GPP) into the category of pregnancy specific dermatoses, citing the fact that GPP is seen specifically in pregnant females. However, it is not clear whether GPP itself is a separate entity or is a variant of generalized pustular psoriasis in which pregnancy acts as a trigger. Due to the unclear classification of GPP we shall discuss it along with psoriasis in the coming chapters. In this chapter we shall discuss the entities which are seen specifically during pregnancy and are classified as pregnancy specific dermatoses as per the existing classification.

Figure 4.

PREGNANCY SPECIFIC DERMATOSES
- Polymorphic eruption of pregnancy (PEP)
- Pemphigoid gestationis (PG)
- Intrahepatic cholestasis of pregnancy (ICP)
- Atopic eruption of pregnancy (AEP)

Some dermatoses have been described in the literature to occur as specific entities during pregnancy. However, there have been reports of the appearance of similar eruptions in the non-pregnant population as well. There are conflicting opinions about placing such dermatoses in the category of pregnancy specific dermatoses. Some less known conditions seen during pregnancy include autoimmune progesterone dermatitis of pregnancy and linear IgM disease of pregnancy. However, there are reports of overlapping similarities and associations with non pregnant states as well. For the sake of clarity and better classification we shall discuss these entities along with pregnancy associated dermatoses in part three of the book as their occurrence is not unique in the context of pregnancy and similar disease states or variants of the same disease are found in the non pregnant population as well. Hence, the existence of these entities as pregnancy specific dermatoses cannot be conclusively established.

References

1. Aronson IK, Kroumpouzos G. Introduction to specific dermatoses. In:Kroumpouzos G, ed. Text Atlas of Obstetric Dermatology. Philadelphia, PA: Lippincott, Williams & Wilkins; 2014. p. 176-179.

2. Sachdeva S. (2008). The dermatoses of pregnancy. Indian journal of dermatology, 53(3), 103–105.

   https://doi.org/10.4103/0019-5154.43203

3. Kroumpouzos G, Cohen LM. Specific dermatoses of pregnancy: an evidence-based systematic review. Am J Obstet Gynecol. 2003 Apr;188(4):1083-92. doi:

   10.1067/mob.2003.129. PMID: 12712115.

4. Lehrhoff S, Pomeranz MK. Specific dermatoses of pregnancy and their treatment. Dermatol Ther. 2013;26:274-284.

5. Holmes RC, Black MM. The specific dermatoses of pregnancy. J Am Acad Dermatol. 1983;8:405-412.

6. Luan L, Han S, Zhang Z, et al. Personal treatment experience for severe generalized pustular psoriasis of pregnancy: Two case reports. Dermatol Ther. 2014;27:174-177.

7. Ambros-Rudolph CM, Müllegger RR, Vaughan-Jones SA, Kerl H, Black MM. The specific dermatoses of pregnancy revisited and reclassified: results of a retrospective two-center study on 505 pregnant patients. J Am Acad Dermatol. 2006 Mar;54(3):395-404. doi: 10.1016/j.jaad.2005.12.012. PMID: 16488288.

Chapter 4

Polymorphic Eruption Of Pregnancy (PEP)

Synonyms: Pruritic Urticarial Papules And Plaques Of Pregnancy (PUPP); Toxemic rash of pregnancy; Toxic erythema of pregnancy

Polymorphic eruption of pregnancy (PEP) is now the most widely accepted terminology for this condition. It is a pregnancy associated benign and reversible skin disorder affecting mainly the primigravida, typically during the third trimester of pregnancy or immediate postpartum period. It presents in the form of severely itchy urticarial lesions, papules and plaques on the abdomen, buttocks and upper thighs often initiating in the area of stretch marks.

Etiopathogenesis

Despite its common occurrence; the etiology is not clear. Because PEP has a predilection towards striae; it is believed that maternal weight gain during pregnancy may cause disruption of the connective tissue in the stretch marks, which may expose an unidentified antigen in the dermis thus triggering an immune response. Increased number of antigen presenting cells and T lymphocytes have also been identified in the lesions of PEP. The predominant occurrence of this condition in first pregnancy supports the neo-antigen theory and development of immune tolerance during subsequent pregnancy. Another theory suggests that fetal DNA itself may act as a neo-antigen. The detection of new antigen can lead to activation of a delayed immune response and consequently may manifest in the form of inflammatory lesions, predominantly involving the abdominal region and the upper thighs where striae are mostly present.

By-products of placental metabolism and hormonal alterations during pregnancy are also attributed as possible factors that can trigger PEP. Increased levels of progesterone hormone and higher expression of progesterone receptors in the skin lesions as compared to the non lesional skin have been demonstrated, thus supporting the role of hormonal modulation. Increased eosinophilic infiltration and association with atopy has also been reported. However, whether atopic eruption of pregnancy is associated with this condition or not remains to be a matter of debate.

Clinical presentation

PEP is one of the most common pregnancy specific dermatoses, more commonly seen in women during their first pregnancy. The rash typically appears during the third trimester or immediate postpartum period and usually undergoes spontaneous resolution after pregnancy. Recurrence during subsequent pregnancy is uncommon and even if it reoccurs; that disease tends to be less severe than the initial episode.

Typically the patients present with urticarial papules on the abdomen, buttocks or upper thighs arising in or around stretch marks which later coalesce to form urticarial plaques. This is followed by a centrifugal spread to the rest of the trunk and extremities. Typically the periumbilical region is spared which can differentiate this condition from other similar dermatoses known as pemphigoid gestationis (PG). Involvement of the face, palms and soles is usually not seen. Mucosal involvement is also not seen. The lesions are often associated with intense itching, however, excoriations are usually not seen. As the name suggests, the lesions may often be polymorphic with the presence of wheals, papules and plaques. Less commonly, target lesions, vesicles and eczematous lesions can also be seen. PEP is broadly divided into three clinical types based on the presentation.

Type 1: Predominantly urticarial papules and plaques.

Type 2: Not urticated papules, plaques or vesicles.

Type3: Mixed Type consisting of both urticarial and non urticarial lesions.

Disease course and prognosis

The skin lesions tend to resolve after six weeks of pregnancy, however, symptoms decrease more quickly after delivery. Some of the lesions may resolve with hyperpigmentation.

Maternal and fetal prognosis usually remains good. Recurrences during subsequent pregnancies are uncommon, however they may occur in less severe form than the primary eruption. Exacerbation of PEP has not been seen during the postpartum period with menstruation or with the use of oral contraceptive pills.

Histopathology

Epidermal changes include acanthosis, orthokeratosis, focal parakeratosis and spongiosis. Vesicles are present in the intra-epidermal region but sometimes may be sub-epidermal. Dermis may show deep and superficial lymphohistiocytic infiltrate with presence of eosinophils. Upper dermal edema is also commonly seen. Direct immunofluorescence study is usually negative and may be used to differentiate it from pemphigoid gestationis.

Differential Diagnosis

Conditions like pemphigoid gestationis should be differentiated from PEP. Sparing of the umbilicus and lesions of PEP favoring the stretch marks are useful differentiators. In case of doubt DIF should be done, which is negative in case of PEP. Enzyme linked immunosorbent assay for the presence of extracellular NC16A domain of BP-180 is usually positive in PG and negative in PEP.

Targetoid lesions seen in PEP should be differentiated from herpes simplex infection, EM and chicken pox. Wheals should be differentiated from those in urticaria and insect bites. Eczematous lesions can be confused with atopic eruption of pregnancy and contact eczemas. Atopic Eruption of Pregnancy (AEP) usually presents early in pregnancy unlike PEP which occurs late in the third trimester. Urticarial lesions which are commonly seen in PEP are not seen in AEP. Patients of AEP often have a history of atopy and recurrences while PEP rarely reoccurs.

Another pruritic disorder in pregnancy known as Intrahepatic Cholestasis of Pregnancy (ICP) usually presents with intense pruritus especially over the palms and soles with secondary excoriations however unlike PEP it lacks primary skin lesions like urticated papules and plaques. The presence of cholestasis, raised blood bile acid levels and recurrence in subsequent pregnancies point towards ICP as these findings are not typically seen in PEP.

Management

Treatment of patients of PEP is predominantly based on the principle of conservative management. The extent of treatment aggression depends on the severity of symptoms and extent of lesions. Topical treatment includes use of emollients preferably containing topical antipruritics like menthol and topical corticosteroids. Oral medications include the use of safer oral antihistamines and short courses of oral steroids if required. Oral prednisolone is usually preferred in case oral steroids are required. Steroids should be used judiciously in the lowest dose required and for the shortest time required. During the lactation period, if steroids are indicated they should be given at least 4 hours before breastfeeding so as to decrease their concentration in the breast milk. Recently, some studies have tried autologous whole blood therapy as a therapeutic modality in PEP which was injected intramuscularly and improvement in disease severity was reported.

References

1. Griffith, C. E.M., & Baker, J. (Eds.). (2016). Rook's Textbook of Dermatology (9th ed., Vol. 3). Willey Blackwell.

2. Ingber, A. (2008). Obstetric Dermatology: A Practical Guide. Springer.

3. Tyler, K. H. (Ed.). (2020). Cutaneous Disorders of Pregnancy. Springer International Publishing.

4. Chouk C, Litaiem N. Pruritic Urticarial Papules And Plaques Of Pregnancy. [Updated 2022 Aug 1]. In: StatPearls [Internet]. Treasure Island (FL): StatPearls Publishing; 2022 Jan. Available from:

   https://www.ncbi.nlm.nih.gov/books/NBK539700

5. Rudolph CM, Al-Fares S, Vaughan-Jones SA, et al. Polymorphic eruption of pregnancy: clinicopathology and potential trigger factors in 181 patients. Br J Dermatol. 2006;154:54–60. [PubMed] [Google Scholar]

6. Powell FC. Pruritic urticarial papules and plaques of pregnancy and multiple pregnancies. J Am Acad Dermatol. 2000;43:730–1. [PubMed] [Google Scholar]

7. Cohen LM, Capeless EL, Krusinski PA, Maloney ME. Pruritic urticarial papules and plaques of pregnancy and its relationship to maternal-fetal weight gain and twin pregnancy. Arch Dernatol. 1989;125:1534–6. [PubMed] [Google Scholar]

8. Elling SV, McKenna P, Powell FC. Pruritic urticarial papules and plaques of pregnancy in twin and triplet pregnancies. J Eur Acad Dermatol Venereol. 2000;14:378–81. [PubMed] [Google Scholar]

9. Pritzier, E. C., & Mikkelsen, C. S. (2012). Polymorphic eruption of pregnancy developing postpartum: 2 case reports. Dermatology reports, 4(1), e7.

   https://doi.org/10.4081/dr.2012.e7

10. Brandão, Pedro & Sousa-Faria, Bárbara & Marinho, Carla & Vieira-Enes, Pedro & Melo, Anabela & Mota, Lurdes. (2016). Polymorphic eruption of pregnancy: Review of literature. Journal of obstetrics and gynaecology : the journal of the Institute of Obstetrics and Gynaecology. 37. 1-4. 10.1080/01443615.2016.1225019.

11. Matz H, Orion E, Wolf R. Pruritic urticarial papules and plaques of pregnancy: polymorphic eruption of pregnancy (PUPPP) Clin Dermatol. 2006;24:105–8. [PubMed] [Google Scholar]

12. Vadakkumpadam MH, Abualiat AS, Sabrah TA. A review of literature of polymorphic eruption of pregnancy. Int J Res Dermatol 2021;7:490-5.

13. Kim EH. Pruritic Urticarial Papules and Plaques of Pregnancy Occurring Postpartum Treated with Intramuscular Injection of Autologous Whole Blood. Case Rep Dermatol. 2017 Jan-Apr;9(1):151-156.

Chapter 5

Pemphigoid Gestationis (PG)

Synonyms : Herpes Gestationis; Gestational Pemphigoid

The term herpes gestation is a misnomer because the disease has no association with herpes viral infection. It is an uncommon, hormonally mediated autoimmune disorder characterized by the presence of intensely itchy urticarial papules and plaques associated with vesiculobullous lesions during pregnancy specially during the second and third trimester.

Etiopathogenesis

Pemphigoid gestationis (PG) is an autoimmune disease characterized by formation of autoantibodies against the non collagenous domain of BP 180 known as NC16A domain. BP 180 is a hemidesmosomal protein found in the umbilical cord and amniotic membrane of the fetus as well as the basement membrane of the mother. The exposure of the maternal immune system to the fetal antigens leads to development of an autoimmune response against the basement membrane structure BP 180 of the maternal basement membrane. This leads to formation of immunoglobulins predominantly of IgG-4 subclass which can cross the placenta. The immune activation leads to infiltration of immune cells especially eosinophils in the basement membrane of the mother, which are the main contributors in disruption of the maternal basement membrane. Association with major histocompatibility complex protein HLA DR3 and HLA DR4 has also been demonstrated. In addition to this, hormonal alterations in pregnancy also contribute to the causation of pemphigoid gestationis. Increased levels of estrogen promotes the production of autoantibodies and serves as an important contributor in the causation. Disease flares can also be seen secondary to the use of oral contraceptive pills and hormonal alterations caused during menstruation.

Clinical presentation

It usually presents in the form of intense pruritus which is followed by development of urticarial rash along with papules and plaques initially located in the periumbilical region and later on spreading centrifugally to the adjoining areas except the face, palms and soles. The urticarial papules and plaques may give rise to vesiculobullous later on. Unlike in PEP, the lesions in pemphigoid gestationis start around the umbilicus and may or may not involve the stretch marks. Mucus membranes are usually spared.

Disease course and prognosis

PG usually affects multigravida females during the second or third trimester of pregnancy. Recurrences usually happen during subsequent pregnancies and are often more severe than previous pregnancies.

The intensity of disease may decrease weeks before delivery followed by an exaggeration immediately after delivery. Following delivery, the lesions start to resolve slowly and the majority of pregnant females become symptom free within the first 6 months after delivery.

Effects on the neonate include appearance of similar lesions resembling maternal lesions at birth which are due to the passage of autoantibodies through placenta to the fetal circulation. It is seen in around 5 to 10 percent of the neonates. However the skin lesions are usually mild and resolve spontaneously within weeks after birth. The occurrence of pemphigoid gestationis is also associated with the higher incidence of prematurity and intrauterine growth retardation, especially in cases with severe disease. Unlike PEP, the risk of recurrence in subsequent pregnancies is very high ranging from one third to one half of the cases. The disease also tends to be more severe and earlier in onset during subsequent pregnancies. Skip pregnancy can also be seen in around 8 percent of cases. PG has also been associated with other autoimmune diseases especially Grave's disease.

Histopathology

Increased infiltration of eosinophils in the dermis along with dermal edema is a common finding in early stages. Later a blister develops with a subepidermal level of split. DIF may show deposition of IgG and C3 along the dermo-epidermal junction. On salt split skin testing, linear deposits of immune reactants are seen on the epidermal side. Enzyme linked immunoassay demonstrates the presence of the NC16A domain of BP 180. Antibody levels correlate with the disease severity and can be used to check the response to treatment.

Differential diagnosis

PG should be differentiated from other pregnancy dermatoses, especially PEP and atopic eruption of pregnancy. Abdominal involvement, intense itching and presence of urticarial papules is common to both PEP and PG. However, the umbilical area is usually spared in PEP and vesicles are not very commonly seen in PEP. DIF may also be needed in doubtful cases to differentiate PG from PEP.

Atopic eruption of pregnancy can be differentiated from PG by a more widespread involvement especially flexural, a pre-existing atopic diathesis, family history and cutaneous xerosis. Other pregnancy related dermatoses like intra hepatic cholestasis of pregnancy, dermatitis herpetiformis, drug eruptions and contact dermatitis should also be kept in mind while diagnosing PG.

Management

Treatment of PG is dependent on the severity of disease. Localized and mild disease can be adequately treated with topical steroids. Itching can be controlled with the use of oral antihistamines. In case of a more widespread or severe disease, oral corticosteroids preferably prednisolone can be added. Lower doses of prednisolone less than 0.5mg / kg / day should ideally be used for acute control of the disease. The dose should be tapered as soon as the disease comes under control, in order to avoid unnecessary side effects of oral steroids. Other therapies like the use of intravenous immunoglobulin, azathioprine, plasma exchange and cyclosporine have been tried in difficult cases.

References

1. Griffith, C. E.M., & Baker, J. (Eds.). (2016). Rook's Textbook of Dermatology (9th ed., Vol. 3). Willey Blackwell.

2. Ingber, A. (2008). Obstetric Dermatology: A Practical Guide. Springer.

3. Tyler, K. H. (Ed.). (2020). Cutaneous Disorders of Pregnancy. Springer International Publishing.

4. Ceryn J., Siekierko A., Skibińska M., Doss N., Narbutt J., & Lesiak A. (2021). Pemphigoid Gestationis - Case Report and Review of Literature. Clinical, cosmetic and investigational dermatology, 14, 665–670.

   https://doi.org/10.2147/CCID.S297520

5. Ambros-Rudolph CM, Müllegger RR, Vaughan-Jones SA, Kerl H, Black MM. The specific dermatoses of pregnancy revisited and reclassified: results of a retrospective two-center study on 505 pregnant patients. J Am Acad Dermatol. 2006;54(3):395–404. doi: 10.1016/j.jaad.2005.12.012

6. Vaughan Jones SA, Hern S, Nelson-Piercy C, Seed PT, Black MM. A prospective study of 200 women with dermatoses of pregnancy correlating clinical findings with hormonal and immunopathological profiles. Br J Dermatol. 1999;141(1):71–81. doi: 10.1046/j.1365-2133.1999.02923.x

7. Lipozenčić J, Ljubojevic S, Bukvić-Mokos Z. Pemphigoid gestationis. Clin Dermatol. 2012;30(1):51–55. doi: 10.1016/j.clindermatol.2011.03.009

8. Huilaja L, Mäkikallio K, Tasanen K. Gestational pemphigoid. Orphanet J Rare Dis. 2014;9:136. doi: 10.1186/s13023-014-0136-2

9. Huilaja L, Mäkikallio K, Sormunen R, Lohi J, Hurskainen T, Tasanen K. Gestational pemphigoid: placental morphology and function. Acta Derm Venereol. 2013;93(1):33–38. doi: 10.2340/00015555-1370

10. Sävervall C, Sand FL, Thomsen SF. Pemphigoid gestationis: current perspectives. Clin Cosmet Investig Dermatol. 2017;10:441–449. doi: 10.2147/CCID.S128144

11. Kumar S, Biswas M, Rajagopal R, Datta S, Narayan B. Successfully treated case of pemphigoid gestationis with post-partum intravenous and oral steroids. J Obstet Gynaecol India. 2014;64(Suppl 1):16-18. doi:10.1007/s13224-013-0408-0

12. Singla A, Shree S, Mehta S. Pregnancy with Pemphigoid Gestationis: A Rare Entity. J Clin Diagn Res. 2016;10(7):QD06-QD7. doi:10.7860/JCDR/2016/19491.8215

Chapter 6

Atopic Eruption of Pregnancy (AEP)

Synonyms: Eczema of pregnancy; Prurigo of pregnancy; Prurigo Gestationis

Atopic eruption of pregnancy is a broad term used to include various pregnancy dermatoses characterized by the presence of itchy, papular and eczematous skin lesions in females often with atopic predisposition. It is a benign dermatosis and usually resolves after pregnancy. It is one of the most common pregnancy dermatoses and accounts for more than half of the pregnancy dermatoses cases. Strong history of atopic diathesis in the patient or family members in the form of allergic rhinitis or asthma can commonly be found.

Etiopathogenesis

AEP is most likely a multifactorial disease. Genetic predisposition associated with immunological changes occurring in pregnancy and contributory factors like environment exposures and abnormal skin barrier, may contribute to the causation of this disease. Pregnancy leads to a shift of immune response from Th1 to Th 2 pathway to prevent rejection of the fetus. This leads to an increased production of Th2 cytokines like interleukin 4 which further contributes to the elevation of IgE levels in the blood. These changes are believed to trigger an inflammatory response in the skin which manifests as atopic eruption of pregnancy.

Clinical presentation

The disease can present itself in the form of exacerbation of preexisting skin lesions or appearance of eczematous lesions de novo. The disease starts early in the course of pregnancy with the majority of the patients presenting within the first two trimesters. AEP can occur in both multi gravida and primary gravida females. AEP is broadly classified into two main types; **E type/ Eczematous type** and **P type/ Papular type**.

Eczematous type is seen in around two-thirds of the cases and is characterized by the presence of scaly erythematous and eczematous skin lesions affecting the atopic sites like the face, neck and the flexural aspect of the upper and lower limbs. These changes can occur in patients already having atopic dermatitis or de novo. Papular type is characterized by the presence of red papules and prurigo-like lesions more on the forearms and the shins. This is often associated with severe cutaneous xerosis.

Disease course and prognosis

The lesions of AEP are usually benign and tend to regress within 3 months after delivery. However in patients with atopic diathesis, disease flares may be seen on and off. Recurrence during subsequent pregnancy are fairly common. As a general rule, AEP is considered to be harmless for both the mother and the child. Pregnancy overall has an exacerbating effect on eczema where in around 50 % of the patients experience worsening while 25% report improvement in symptoms of eczema.

Histopathology

The findings in histopathology are often non-specific resembling any dermatitis. Epidermal changes include acanthosis, hyperkeratosis, parakeratosis and spongiosis. Dermis shows perivascular lymphohistiocytic infiltrate along with eosinophils. Accompanying dermal edema may also be seen. Immunofluorescence studies are usually negative.

Differential diagnosis

Pruritus gravidarum which is a benign physiological pruritus seen in pregnancy, is characterized by the presence of isolated excoriations without any primary lesions that must be differentiated from atopic eruption of pregnancy. Dryness of the skin may otherwise also be seen in pregnancy, especially on the lower legs but should not be misdiagnosed as AEP in absence of eczematous itchy lesions.

Other pregnancy dermatoses like polymorphic eruption of pregnancy, intrahepatic cholestasis of pregnancy and pemphigoid gestationis should also be excluded. Exogenous dermatitis which has a history of external exposure should also be excluded. Drug induced eruptions and insect bite hypersensitivity also need to be excluded.

Management

Laboratory investigations may reveal variable amounts of eosinophilia and raised IgE levels in some patients.

Treatment will depend upon the distribution and severity of disease. Mild disease with a localized extent can be treated with liberal use of emollients and judicious use of topical steroids. Severe cases would often require a short course of oral corticosteroids. Whenever needed, prednisolone should be the preferred oral corticosteroid. The use of oral corticosteroids in the first trimester of pregnancy should be avoided to prevent any deleterious effects of steroids on organogenesis and fetal development. Symptomatic control of pruritus can be achieved with the use of oral antihistamines. Narrowband UVB light is another safe and non-invasive therapeutic modality in pregnancy. Secondary superinfections like folliculitis, impetigo and eczema herpeticum should be treated with topical and oral antibiotics or antivirals. In refractory cases; if necessary oral cyclosporine may be considered keeping in view its side effect profile on the fetus and the mother including maternal hypertension and renal side effects.

References

1. Ambros-Rudolph CM, Jones SV. Atopic eruption in pregnancy. Ambros-Rudolph CM, Edwards L, Lynch PJ, Editors. 3rd edn. In: Obstetric and Gynecologic Dermatology. Mosby Elsevier. 2008; 65-72.

2. Griffith, C. E.M., & Baker, J. (Eds.). (2016). Rook's Textbook of Dermatology (9th ed., Vol. 3). Willey Blackwell.

3. Ingber, A. (2008). Obstetric Dermatology: A Practical Guide. Springer.

4. Tyler, K. H. (Ed.). (2020). Cutaneous Disorders of Pregnancy. Springer International Publishing.

5. Ingber A. Atopic Eruption of Pregnancy. J Eur Acad Dermatol Venereol. 2010 ; 24: 984.

6. Savervall C, Sand FL, Thomsen SF. Dermatological Diseases Associated with Pregnancy: Pemphigoid Gestationis, Polymorphic Eruption of Pregnancy, Intrahepatic Cholestasis of Pregnancy, and Atopic Eruption of Pregnancy. Dermatol Res Pract. 2015;2015:979635. doi:10.1155/2015/979635

7. Roth M. M. Pregnancy dermatoses: diagnosis, management, and controversies. American Journal of Clinical Dermatology. 2011;12(1):25–41. doi: 10.2165/11532010-000000000-00000.

8. Di Carlo A, Amon E, Gardner M, Barr S, Ott K. Eczema herpeticum in pregnancy and neonatal herpes infection. Obstet Gynecol. 2008; 112: 455-457.

9. Koutroulis I, Papoutsis J, Kroumpouzos G. Atopic dermatitis in pregnancy: current status and challenges. Obstet Gynecol Surv. 2011; 66: 654-663.

10. Kar S, Krishnan A, Preetha K, Mohankar A. A review of antihistamines used during pregnancy. J Pharmacol Pharmacother. 2012; 3: 105-108.

11. Trønnes H, WilcoxAJ, Markestad T, et al. Associations of maternal atopic diseases with adverse pregnancy outcomes: A national cohort study. Paediatr Perinat Epidemiol. 2014;28:489-497.

12. Massone C, Cerroni L, Heidrun N, Brunasso AMG, Nunzi E, Gulia A, et al. Histopathological diagnosis of atopic eruption of pregnancy and polymorphic eruption of pregnancy: a study on 41 cases. Am J Dermatopathol. 2014;36(10):812–21.

13. Rudder M, Lefkowitz EG, Ruhama T, Firoz E. A review of pruritus in pregnancy. Obstetric Medicine. 2021;14(4):204-210. doi:10.1177/1753495X20985366

Chapter 7

Intrahepatic Cholestasis of Pregnancy (ICP)

Synonyms: Pruritus gravidarum; Obstetric Cholestasis; Jaundice of pregnancy

Intrahepatic Cholestasis of pregnancy (ICP) is a pregnancy dermatoses associated with generalized itching without any primary skin lesions and the presence of secondary excoriations only. It is usually seen during the second half of pregnancy. Some authors differentiate pruritus gravidarum as a benign skin condition characterized by pruritus and caused by physiological and biochemical alteration during pregnancy in the absence of any specific dermatoses. ICP on the other hand is defined as a more severe disease of intense itching, excoriations and raised bile acid levels.

Etiopathogenesis

It is believed to be a multifactorial disease with genetic, environment and hormonal influences contributing to the causation. Genetic factors include the increased occurrence of ICP in 1st degree relatives and the reported mutation in the genes ABC B4 and ABC B 11 which have been linked with ICP.

Hormonal factors include the increased levels of estrogen hormone in pregnancy which impair the excretion of bilirubin leading to cholestasis.

Environmental factors include decreased sunlight exposure leading to low levels of vitamin D and low intake of antioxidants like selenium in the patients.

Clinical presentation

ICP is seen to develop during the second half of pregnancy and it tends to resolve within a few weeks after delivery. Intense generalized pruritus more so on the face, palms and soles is the hallmark of ICP. Secondary excoriations are often seen with the absence of any primary skin lesions. The itching is more pronounced at night and the patients may experience disturbance in sleep. Other associated findings of cholestasis like icterus, loss of appetite, lethargy, yellowish urine and clay coloured stools may be seen. On examination the liver may be enlarged and tender.

Disease course and prognosis

ICP can be associated with significant fetal morbidity. Fetal outcomes in the form of preterm birth, abortion and fetal distress have been reported. Severity of disease directly correlates with severity of complications seen in the fetus. Fetal monitoring is done to identify early signs of fetal distress. Abnormal coagulation caused by liver function derangement and vitamin K deficiency can lead to maternal and fetal hemorrhage. Sequels of ICP during childhood include high fasting insulin levels and more predisposition to obesity. Mothers having ICP had a higher incidence of hepatic complications like cholecystitis and hepatitis

C. ICP tends to recur in almost two third of subsequent pregnancies with varying degrees of severity.

Histopathology

Biopsy of the skin reveals non-specific changes.

Differential diagnosis

Pregnancy dermatoses like atopic eruption of pregnancy, polymorphic eruption of pregnancy and pemphigus gestationis should be differentiated from ICP. Absence of any primary skin lesions and elevated bile acid levels in the blood are hallmark of ICP.

Hepatic disorders like viral hepatitis, obstructive jaundice, drug induced hepatitis and alcoholic liver disease should be ruled out.

Management

Elevated bile acid levels of more than 10 micromol/liter in a pregnant female is diagnostic of ICP. Severity of ICP can also be determined based on the blood levels of bile acids. Total bile acid level of less than 40 micromol/liter is considered as mild whereas levels more than that are considered as severe ICP. Adverse fetal outcome is unlikely if the total bile acid levels stay below 40 micromol/l. Liver enzymes can be elevated as well but usually not more than ten times the upper normal limit. Direct bilirubin levels are usually normal or slightly elevated. Continuation of pruritus after delivery and persistence of deranged liver functions should trigger the doctor to think about other hepatic disorders. Sometimes ultrasonography to rule out biliary tract obstruction is required. Monitoring of liver transaminases can help to determine the response to treatment.

Treatment of ICP is aimed at symptomatic control of itching. General measures like rest and a low fat diet should be advised. Patients should be counseled about the temporary nature of the disease and that the disease usually resolves after childbirth. Mild disease can be dealt with the use of moisturizer containing antipruritic preparation like menthol or calamine. Oral preparations containing silymarin and S adenosyl Methionine have shown good effect in controlling pruritus in mild cases of ICP. Some practitioners recommend terminating the pregnancy at 37 weeks of gestation in severe cases in order to minimize risk to the fetus. Ultraviolet B is another safe and non-invasive modality which has been used in treatment of ICP.

Ursodeoxycholic acid is considered the cornerstone of drug therapy in ICP. It is commonly used in the dose of 300 mg BD to 300 mg QID. Ursodeoxycholic acid not only reduces the bile acid levels in the maternal serum but also reduces the total bile acid levels in the cord blood and amniotic sac. It acts by decreasing the biliary secretion of bile acids and also has a protective action towards hepatocyte injury caused by toxic levels of bile acids. Another bile acid sequestrant known as cholestyramine has also been used in ICP. However, ursodeoxycholic acid is safer, more efficacious and more rapidly acting.

References

1. Griffith, C. E.M., & Baker, J. (Eds.). (2016). Rook's Textbook of Dermatology (9th ed., Vol. 3). Willey Blackwell.

2. Ingber, A. (2008). Obstetric Dermatology: A Practical Guide. Springer.

3. Tyler, K. H. (Ed.). (2020). Cutaneous Disorders of Pregnancy. Springer International Publishing.

4. Pillarisetty LS, Sharma A. Pregnancy Intrahepatic Cholestasis. [Updated 2022.Jun 12]. In: StatPearls [Internet]. Treasure Island (FL): StatPearls Publishing; 2022 Jan-. Available from: https://www.ncbi.nlm.nih.gov/books/NBK551503/

5. Ghosh S, Chaudhuri S. Intra-hepatic cholestasis of pregnancy: A comprehensive review. Indian J Dermatol 2013;58:327

6. Geenes V, Williamson C. Intrahepatic cholestasis of pregnancy. World J Gastroenterol. 2009;15(17):2049-2066. doi:10.3748/wjg.15.2049

7. Piechota J, Jelski W. Intrahepatic Cholestasis in Pregnancy: Review of the Literature. J Clin Med. 2020;9(5):1361. Published 2020 May 6. doi:10.3390/jcm9051361

8. Roncaglia N, Arreghini A, Locatelli A, Bellini P, Andreotti C, Ghidini A. Obstetric cholestasis: outcome with active management. Eur J Obstet Gynecol Reprod Biol. 2002;100(2):167–70.

9. Laifer SA, Stiller RJ, Siddiqui DS, Dunston-Boone G, Whetham JC. Ursodeoxycholic acid for the treatment of intrahepatic cholestasis of pregnancy. J Matern Fetal Med. 2001;10(2):131–5.

10. Lo TK, Lau WL, Lam HS, Leung WC, Chin RK. Obstetric cholestasis in Hong Kong--local experience with eight consecutive cases. Hong Kong Med J (Xianggang yi xue za zhi). 2007;13(5):387–91.

11. Gardiner FW, McCuaig R, Arthur C, Carins T, Morton A, Laurie J, et al. The prevalence and pregnancy outcomes of intrahepatic cholestasis of pregnancy: a retrospective clinical audit review. Obstet Med. 2019;12(3):123–8.

12. Arora S, Huria A, Goel P, Kaur J, Dubey S. Maternal and fetal outcome in intrahepatic cholestasis of pregnancy at tertiary care institute of North India. Indian J Med Sci 2021;73:335-9.

13. Ambros-Rudolph CM, Glatz M, Trauner M, Kerl H, Müllegger RR. The Importance of Serum Bile Acid Level Analysis and Treatment With Ursodeoxycholic Acid in Intrahepatic Cholestasis of Pregnancy: A Case Series From Central Europe. Arch Dermatol. 2007;143(6):757–762.

doi:10.1001/archderm.143.6.757

Part 3

Pregnancy Associated Dermatoses

Chapter 8

Inflammatory Dermatoses In Pregnancy

Atopic dermatitis

Atopic dermatitis is an itchy inflammatory dermatoses with an increased prevalence in developed nations.

Etiopathogenesis

It is considered to be a multifactorial disease involving genetic predisposition, immunological and environmental factors. There is also a shift in adaptive immune response to words Th2 pathway in atopic dermatitis. This leads to overexpression of the Th2 cytokines and high levels of serum IgE has been demonstrated. Pregnancy itself being Th2 predominant state results in exacerbation of pre-existing atopic dermatitis. A similar flare up of atopic dermatitis is seen during menstruation which suggests the effect of increased sex hormones during pregnancy especially progesterone levels which contributes towards exacerbation of atopic dermatitis in pregnancy.

Clinical presentation

Atopic dermatitis during pregnancy presents with lesions similar to atopic dermatitis seen otherwise with predominant flexural distribution and involvement of face, neck, flexural aspect of upper and lower limbs especially fossae and the inframammary region. Hands and feet are also commonly involved. Lesions can vary from oozy and eczematous to dry and cracked lesions. Other findings including keratosis pilaris, hyperlinear palms and lichenification can also be seen. The areola and nipple skin may also be cracked and eczematised which can pose a problem during breastfeeding.

Disease course and prognosis

Atopic dermatitis during pregnancy is not known to cause adverse fetal or maternal outcome; the condition otherwise is benign and does not affect the outcome or plan of delivery. However mothers suffering from atopic dermatitis have an increased risk of atopy in the child.

Management

Laboratory investigations may reveal eosinophilia and raised serum IgE levels. TLC may be raised in presence of a secondary co-infection.

Treatment of atopic dermatitis includes liberal use of emollients which is the backbone of therapy in atopic dermatitis. Patients are advised to use mild cleansers or soap substitutes to avoid excessive drying of the skin. Mild to moderate potency topical steroids can also be used in the initial phases of treatment for subsidence of skin lesions. Topical steroids are pregnancy category C drugs and are considered safer than oral corticosteroids. While using topical steroids, the patient should be instructed to clean the nipple area before breastfeeding. Topical antibiotics like mupirocin and fusidic acid cream are safe to use in pregnancy in cases of superadded skin infections. Topical calcineurin inhibitors like tacrolimus are pregnancy category C drugs however extensive data regarding the safety of calcineurin inhibitors in pregnancy is not available. Presumably, due to the large molecular size of the drug the systemic absorption is believed to be minimal. In case of non responsive cases narrowband UVB can also be used as a safe second line option. Oral treatment may include use of antihistamines to check pruritus and sleep disturbance. A short course of oral steroids should be used only if the disease is uncontrolled with the above mentioned modalities. Oral corticosteroids should be avoided especially during the first trimester of pregnancy.

Oral immunosuppressants like cyclosporine which is the pregnancy category C can cross the placenta. However animal studies have shown that fetal toxicity occurs only when very high doses of cyclosporine were instituted to the mother. Before prescribing cyclosporine a risk-benefit analysis of the drug should be kept in mind. Cyclosporine however should not be used during breastfeeding as it is secreted in the breast milk.

Azathioprine is the FDA pregnancy category D drug. It is seen to cross the placenta and has been reported to be associated with adverse pregnancy outcomes like preterm delivery, small for gestation babies and low birth weight. There are inadequate studies to assess safety of azathioprine in pregnant females with atopic dermatitis. Moreover, azathioprine is also secreted in breast milk and should be avoided during breastfeeding. Therefore azathioprine should only be considered when all other safer options have been exhausted.

Dupilumab is a biological agent which has shown to be efficacious in atopic dermatitis however the data to assess it's safety in pregnant females is lacking and until adequate data is available dupilumab is not recommended to be used in pregnant females. Certain agents which should not be used in atopic dermatitis of pregnancy include methotrexate because of its teratogenic effects. It should be stopped at least 3 months prior to planning conception. Mycophenolate mofetil is another category D drug which should be avoided because of increasing evidence of its teratogenicity. PUVA should also be avoided as it involves the use of oral psoralen.

Allergic contact dermatitis

Allergic contact dermatitis is predominantly a delayed hypersensitivity reaction to an exogenous allergen. It appears to be a predominantly Th1 pathway mediated immune response with overexpression of Type 1 cytokines like interferon gamma, interleukin 2 and TNF alpha.

Since pregnancy involves a shift of immune response from the Th1 to Th2 pathway, conditions like allergic contact dermatitis which are Th1 mediated should decrease in intensity. Also during the pregnancy there is overexpression of IL-10 which is known to block the effector pathway in allergic contact dermatitis. However it is difficult to quantify in practice regarding the improvement of allergic contact dermatitis in pregnancy if any, due to conflicting data and inadequate understanding about the effect of pregnancy on allergic contact dermatitis. Flare-ups of allergic contact dermatitis have been seen in cases during the postpartum period possibly due to the reversal of immune response and predominance of Th1 immune response during the postpartum period.

Management of allergic contact dermatitis remains more or less same during pregnancy as it is in other patients. However, the treatment should be more on the conservative side and efforts should be made to ensure fair usage of drugs in order to avoid any deleterious effects of drug therapy on the mother or the fetus.

Psoriasis

Psoriasis is a chronic inflammatory dermatoses characterized by the presence of scaly red papules and plaques which are well defined with a predominant extensoral distribution. These lesions characteristically have lamellar silvery scales. It can be a limited disease with the presence of few lesions or can be widespread. Other sites like the scalp, nails and joints can also be involved.

Etiopathogenesis

It is believed that progesterone hormone has a direct effect on epidermal cells through progesterone receptors located on the keratinocytes. Psoriasis is known to involve the Th1 pathway. However in pregnancy there is a shift from the Th1 to Th2 pathway which may explain the improvement seen in pregnant females. Estrogen on the other hand has shown to augment B cell immunity and suppress T cell mediated immune response. This itself may have an inhibitory effect on the pathogenesis of psoriasis.

Effect of psoriasis on pregnancy

The data regarding the effect of psoriasis on pregnancy is inadequate and conflicting. Some previous studies have shown that the incidence of abortion, low birth weight, prematurity and cesarean delivery is more in patients having psoriasis. Whereas recent studies have shown no such association. There is a possibility of adverse maternal and fetal outcomes in cases of severe psoriasis. The cases of severe psoriasis should be adequately monitored for maternal and fetal health so that timely intervention can be instituted. There has been evidence of placental insufficiency, intrauterine growth retardation and fetal distress in cases of severe psoriasis.

Effect of pregnancy on psoriasis

Females having psoriasis are usually seen to improve during pregnancy. Around 50% of psoriatic pregnant females report improvement in the lesions, whereas 25% of the patients report stabilization of psoriasis. Exacerbation of psoriasis is seen in only one fourth of the cases. Psoriasis can however flare up during the postpartum period.

Management

The treatment of psoriasis in pregnancy should aim towards minimizing the adverse effects on the fetus and the mother. In cases of mild to moderate psoriasis; no active intervention may be needed as in most of the cases psoriasis tends to decrease in aggression after pregnancy starts. In cases of severe disease, treatment should ideally be started before conception so as to decrease the intensity of the disease and to minimize the adverse effects of psoriasis on the outcome of pregnancy.

Initial treatment of psoriasis in pregnancy should start with the use of moisturizers and mild to moderate potency steroids. Treatment with topical agents is usually sufficient in cases with limited distribution of the disease involving less than 10% of body surface area. In cases who do not respond adequately to the topical line of therapy or where the maximum safe limit of topical steroids is exceeded; narrow band UVB light becomes a reasonable and safer option to be used. In patients where narrowband UVB is used, supplemental folic acid should be given in the form of oral tablets because long term use of NBUVB leads to deficiency of folic acid in the body. The deficiency of folic acid during pregnancy can be associated with neural tube defects in the fetus. Oral corticosteroids are conventionally not recommended in cases of psoriasis. They can however be used if required in cases of generalized pustular psoriasis in pregnancy.

In refractory cases of plaque psoriasis in pregnancy, oral and parenteral agents which can be used with caution include cyclosporine for short-term rescue therapy and biologicals like anti TNF alpha inhibitors. However, risk benefit analysis should be done before these agents are started. Biological agents are category B drugs in pregnancy, however, their safety data is lacking. When they are to be used, older biologicals which have some amount of data like etanercept should be preferred.

Drugs which should not be used in pregnancy associated with psoriasis include methotrexate which is a pregnancy category X drug and is highly teratogenic. PUVA therapy should also be avoided as it includes the use of oral psoralens. Another drug which should be avoided in pregnant psoriatic patients is acitretin.

The patient has to be off the drug for at least three years before planning pregnancy. Topical agents which are conventionally used in psoriasis but should be avoided in pregnant psoriatic patients include topical retinoids, topical salicylic acid, coal tar dithranol and vitamin D analogues.

Generalized Pustular psoriasis of Pregnancy (GPP)

Also known as Impetigo herpetiformis, it is a variant of pustular psoriasis seen in pregnant females. It is an uncommon disease and unlike plaque psoriasis in pregnancy, it often occurs in patients who have no history of psoriasis in the past. The condition often resolves after delivery. It is because of this reason that some authors prefer to place it in the category of pregnancy specific dermatoses. The disease should more appropriately be called GPP as the term Impetigo herpetiformis is a misnomer since the disease is neither a bacterial infection (impetigo) nor is it associated with herpes virus.

Etiopathogenesis

The exact cause of GPP is still not known. However, hormone mediated immune modulation is believed to play a role in the pathogenesis of GPP. Other factors like decreased levels of serum calcium and hypoparathyroidism may also contribute to the causation of the disease. GPP which is now believed to be a variant of pustular psoriasis is associated with a more significant role of IL-1 and IL-36 which promote neutrophil chemotaxis responsible form pustule formation.

Some studies have reported mutations involving the genes coding for the antagonists of IL-1 subtype receptors like IL36RN in patients of GPP.

Clinical presentation

Generalized pustular psoriasis of pregnancy can appear during any trimester of pregnancy. It presents in the form of diffuse background erythema studded with numerous pinpoint pustules which can be seen arranged in a concentric or annular or circinate arrangement. These pustules may often coalesce to form lakes of pus. Later on, dried areas of pus may give rise to central crusting. The skin lesions are predominantly present on the periumbilical, intertriginous areas and flexures but may also involve the trunk and limbs. Palms and soles are usually not affected. The disease can be associated with constitutional symptoms in the form of fever, nausea, vomiting, malaise diarrhea, muscle aches and CNS symptoms like delirium. Hypocalcemia may manifest clinically in the form of tetany.

GPP classically develops during the second half of pregnancy and undergoes remission after delivery. Recurrences in subsequent pregnancies are seen to occur early and episodes are usually more severe. Fetal adverse outcomes in the form of stillbirths, intrauterine death and congenital abnormalities have been reported.

Differential diagnosis

Diseases which can present with pustular or bullous eruptions like candidiasis, AGEP, bullous impetigo, pemphigoid gestationis, polymorphic eruption of pregnancy, subcorneal pustular dermatoses, dermatitis herpetiformis etc should be differentiated from GPP.

Histopathology

Skin biopsy of the patient of GPP shows findings similar to that of pustular psoriasis. Epidermis shows parakeratosis, elongation of rete ridges along with numerous spongiform pustules of kogoj. Immunofluorescence studies are negative.

Management

Laboratory investigations may detect an elevated leukocyte count, elevated erythrocyte sedimentation rate; blood electrolytes along with serum calcium levels should also be evaluated to rule out hypocalcemia.

The disease can have fatal consequences for the mother if left untreated. Thus early diagnosis and treatment is a must. The treatment is usually tapered after disease is controlled and often continued in lower doses till delivery as GPP tends to flare up on discontinuation.

Urticaria

Introduction

Urticaria is a transient dermatoses characterized by well described raised itchy, erythematous and evanescent lesions known as wheals. Wheals arise because of the increased vascular permeability and vasodilation leading to edema of the papillary dermis. Urticaria is further classified into acute and chronic subtypes. Urticaria which persists for more than 6 weeks is termed as chronic whereas urticaria lasting for less than six weeks is called acute urticaria. Urticaria may sometimes be associated with a condition known as angioedema. It is caused due to swelling of the deeper dermis and subcutis or the submucosal tissue often presenting with swelling involving the areas of lax skin like periorbital areas, lips and genitalia. Mucosal sites like pharynx and larynx may also be involved which sometimes may be life threatening if it causes obstruction of the airway.

Pregnancy and Urticaria

Pregnancy is characterized by a higher than usual incidence of urticaria with or without angioedema. Increased incidence of physical urticaria, especially pressure urticaria has been reported in association with pregnancy. Multiple factors like hormonal alterations, medications and extrinsic exposures during pregnancy can trigger urticaria. Urticaria may be secondary to external antigenic exposure or due to allergic sensitization caused by endogenous hormones especially progesterone. Besides pregnancy, exacerbations and flare-ups of urticarial episodes have also been reported during the menstrual periods signifying an underlying hormonal influence. High levels of endogenous progesterone have also been linked to the occurrence of anaphylaxis in some pregnant females. Urticaria in pregnancy is not known to cause adverse effects on the fetus or mother neither does it affect the fertility in females.

Differential Diagnosis

Urticaria in pregnancy needs to be differentiated from early pre bullous urticarial lesions of the pemphigoid gestationis. Another disease which can closely resemble urticaria of pregnancy is PEP.

Management

The principle of management of urticaria in pregnancy remains the same as in non pregnant cases. Judicious use of safe antihistamines and topical antipruritic lotions is sufficient in most of the cases of urticaria associated with pregnancy. First generation antihistamines like chlorpheniramine have good safety data in pregnancy. Among second generation antihistamines loratadine and cetirizine are usually preferred. Flare-ups of urticaria associated with pregnancy often subside or decrease in intensity once the pregnancy is over.

Erythema nodosum (EN)

Etiopathogenesis

Erythema nodosum is believed to be a type 3 hypersensitivity reaction mediated by the deposition of an immune complex in the dermis and subcutaneous tissue manifesting clinically in the form of erythematous and tender nodules. The immune response may be secondary to a variety of causative factors including infections which can be bacterial, viral, fungal or parasitic. In the Indian context; tuberculosis is one of the most common and important infections other than streptococcal infections. EN may also be triggered by drugs like sulfonamides, oral contraceptives and iodides. It may also occur secondary to various disorders like sarcoidosis, ulcerative colitis, behcet's disease etc. Pregnancy is also known to be associated with erythema nodosum. The very fact that erythema nodosum can be precipitated by the use of oral contraceptive pills and pregnancy signifies the underlying hormonal influence of pregnancy on the occurrence of erythema nodosum. The hormonal changes during pregnancy are well established in causation of erythema nodosum. Some authors also attribute the role of fetal antigens in triggering the immune response of erythema nodosum.

Clinical presentation

It is a cutaneous condition characterized by the appearance of tender, raised, red inflammatory nodules which are localized predominantly on the extensor surfaces of the upper and lower limbs most characteristically seen on the shins. The condition is usually self-limiting and the lesions heal with characteristic color changes followed by hyper pigmentation. The appearance of lesions may be associated with constitutional symptoms in the form of fever, malaise, arthralgias, myalgias and pedal edema. It is predominantly seen in the female population. Erythema nodosum associated with pregnancy usually develops during the first trimester or around the time of delivery.

Histopathology

EN is characterized by the presence of septal panniculitis along with the characteristic radial meischer's granulomas.

Management

Erythema nodosum is a self limiting condition and in most of the cases the treatment should be based on a symptomatic approach. General measures like bed rest, use of compression stockings and foot and elevation should be advised. Medications like paracetamol which are safe in pregnancy can be advised for their analgesic and anti-inflammatory properties. Erythema nodosum in pregnancy is not known to cause any adverse fetal or maternal complications.

References

1. Griffith, C. E.M., & Baker, J. (Eds.). (2016). Rook's Textbook of Dermatology (9th ed., Vol. 3). Willey Blackwell.

2. Ingber, A. (2008). Obstetric Dermatology: A Practical Guide. Springer.

3. Tyler, K. H. (Ed.). (2020). Cutaneous Disorders of Pregnancy. Springer International Publishing.

4. Sachdeva S. The dermatoses of pregnancy. Indian J Dermatol 2008;53:103-5

5. Kumari R, Jaisankar T J, Thappa DM. A clinical study of skin changes in pregnancy. Indian J Dermatol Venereol Leprol 2007;73:141

6. Stefaniak, A.A., Pereira, M.P., Zeidler, C. et al. Pruritus in Pregnancy. Am J Clin Dermatol 23, 231–246 (2022). https://doi.org/10.1007/s40257-021-00668-7

7. Koutroulis I, Papoutsis J, Koumpouzos G. Atopic dermatitis in pregnancy: Current status and challenges. Obstet Gynecol Surv. 2011;66: 654-663.

8. Anita Puri, Anisha Sethi, Karan Jit Pal Singh Puri, Anmol Sharma, Correlation of nipple eczema in pregnancy with atopic dermatitis in Northern India: a study of 100 cases, Anais Brasileiros de Dermatologia, Volume 94, Issue 5, 2019,

9. Chi C-C, Mayon-White RT, Wojnarowska FT. Safety of topical corticosteroids in pregnancy: a population-based cohort study. J Invest Dermatol 2011;131:884–91.

10. Bonamonte D, Foti C, Antelmi AR et al (2005) Nickel contact allergy and menstrual cycle.Contact Dermatitis 52:309–313

11. Murase JE, Chan KK, Garite TJ et al (2005) Hormonal effect on psoriasis in pregnancy and postpartum. Arch Dermatol 141:601–606

12. Raychaudhuri SP, Navare T, Gross J et al (2003) Clinical course of psoriasis during pregnancy. Int J Dermatol 42:518–520

13. McHugh NJ, Laurent MR (1989) The effect of pregnancy on the onset of psoriatic arthritis. Br J Rheumatol 28:50–52

14. Namazi N, Dadkhahfar S. Impetigo Herpetiformis: Review of Pathogenesis, Complication, and Treatment. Dermatol Res Pract. 2018;2018:5801280. Published 2018 Apr 4. doi:10.1155/2018/5801280

15. Chang S. E., Kim H. H., Choi J. H., et al. Impetigo herpetiformis followed by generalized pustular psoriasis: more evidence of same disease entity. International Journal of Dermatology. 2003;42(9):754–755

16. Fouda U. M., Fouda R. M., Ammar H. M., Salem M., El Darouti M. Impetigo herpetiformis during the puerperium triggered by secondary hypoparathyroidism: A case report. Cases Journal. 2009;2(12, article no. 9338) doi: 10.1186/1757-1626-2-9338.

17. Puig L., Barco D., Alomar A. Treatment of psoriasis with anti-TNF drugs during pregnancy: Case report and review of the literature. Dermatology. 2010;220(1):71–76. doi: 10.1159/000262284.

18. Bozdag K., Ozturk S., Ermete M. A case of recurrent impetigo herpetiformis treated with systemic corticosteroids and narrowband UVB. Cutaneous and Ocular Toxicology. 2012;31(1):67–69. doi: 10.3109/15569527.2011.602035.

19. Gao Q, -Q, Xi M, -R, Yao Q: Impetigo Herpetiformis during Pregnancy: A Case Report and Literature Review. Dermatology 2013;226:35-40. doi: 10.1159/000346578

20. Kocatürk E, Podder I, Zenclussen AC, et al. Urticaria in Pregnancy and Lactation. Front Allergy. 2022;3:892673. Published 2022 Jul 7. doi:10.3389/falgy.2022.89267

21. Källén B. Use of antihistamine drugs in early pregnancy and delivery outcome. J Matern Fetal Neonatal Med 2002;11(3):146–52.

22. Pérez-Garza DM, Chavez-Alvarez S, Ocampo-Candiani J, Gomez-Flores M. Erythema Nodosum: A Practical Approach and Diagnostic Algorithm. Am J Clin Dermatol. 2021;22(3):367-378. doi:10.1007/s40257-021-00592-w

23. Acosta KA, HaverMC, Kelly B. Etiology and therapeutic management of erythema nodosum during pregnancy: An update. Am J Clin Dermatol. 2013;14:215-222.

24. Salvatore MA. Erythema nodosum, estrogens, and pregnancy. Arch Dermatol. 1980;116:557.

Chapter 9

Autoimmune Connective Tissue Disorders In Pregnancy

Autoimmune connective tissue disorders in pregnancy include a wide range of conditions like lupus erythematosus, dermatomyositis, systemic sclerosis, Sjogren's syndrome etc. We shall discuss the conditions here which are relevant in the context of pregnancy.

Lupus Erythematosus (LE)

Introduction

Lupus erythematosus is a broad term used for a spectrum of presentation based on the nature of the disease and its aggression. It is divided into chronic, subacute and acute types. Chronic lupus erythematosus comprises Discoid LE and other uncommon subtypes like tumid lupus, lupus panniculitis, chilblain lupus etc. Classic LE known as discoid LE presents in the form of coin shaped erythematous to plaques with well defined borders and fine adherent scales.

Deposition of keratin in dilated follicular openings presents as a ***tin tack sign*** in the form of horny projections on the undersurface of scale, when examined on removal. The sub acute type of LE known as SCLE presents with annular and polycyclic lesions or papulosquamous lesions predominantly distributed on the photo exposed areas. The acute variant of LE known as ACLE is less common but the most severe variant of lupus erythematosus. It can present in a localized distribution in the form of malar rash or can be more widespread in the form of diffuse maculopapular rash or its variants which is often more severe. The types of lupus erythematosus are not independent of each other and a significant overlap can be seen in many cases. The degree of systemic involvement is least with chronic type and maximum with acute type.

Disease course and prognosis

Lupus erythematosus is predominantly seen in females. The most common age group in females is of the reproductive age group. It is conventionally believed that systemic lupus erythematosus being a Th2 mediated disease should worsen in pregnancy. Around 50% of SLE patients report exacerbation during pregnancy. However, reports of improvement in SLE during pregnancy as well as stabilization of the disease are also present. Thus no general statement regarding the effect of pregnancy on lupus erythematosus can be made.

Increase in the activity of lupus erythematosus during pregnancy, if present is usually not very severe. Exacerbations are usually seen during the third trimester of pregnancy and in the postpartum period. Pre-pregnancy severity of lupus erythematosus also determines the exaggeration seen during the course of pregnancy.

Severe LE in pregnancy is associated with adverse outcomes for both mother and fetus which includes a higher incidence of preeclampsia, thrombotic episodes, preterm delivery, spontaneous abortion and intrauterine growth retardation. Fertility however is not generally affected. Infertility may sometimes develop in patients of LE secondary to the drugs used in treatment of lupus erythematosus like cyclophosphamide which is known to be gonadotoxic. A good prognostic factor is the attainment of remission in disease activity at least 3 months or ideally more than 6 months before conception. Bad prognostic factors for pregnancy outcome in cases of lupus erythematosus include hypertension, active state of lupus erythematosus during pregnancy, positive anticardiolipin antibodies and Ro/La antibodies, active treatment with corticosteroids and immunosuppressants during pregnancy, systemic involvement and patients of non white race. Cases of lupus erythematosus who had only cutaneous involvement had a better prognosis as compared to cases of systemic lupus erythematosus.

Clinical presentation

The most common manifestation of lupus erythematosus in pregnancy includes flare up of the rash and joint pains. Sometimes, renal and hematological manifestations also occur during pregnancy. Other cutaneous findings commonly seen in these patients include cutaneous rash (localized or diffuse), oral and nasal ulcerations, raynaud's phenomenon, photosensitivity and hair loss. Cutaneous rash can present as localized malar rash or generalized photosensitive rash in acute cases. Chronic LE can present with discoid lesions while subacute LE can present with annular or polycyclic or papulosquamous rash. Many cases initially present with only painful vasculitic lesions of the fingers and toes.

Neonatal lupus erythematosus

Neonatal lupus erythematosus may be seen in the newborn babies of mothers who commonly are anti Ro/La antibody positive. The neonate can present with skin lesions resembling subacute lupus or with congenital heart block. Hepatic and hematological abnormality can also be associated. Cutaneous rash in the neonate is usually photo distributed on the face and scalp. The rash may either be annular, polycyclic or papulosquamous and is often triggered after photo exposure. The condition in neonates is fortunately self limiting and often resolves on its own as the pathogenic autoantibodies get depleted from neonatal circulation.

Management

Prepregnancy management would include optimizing the treatment regime so as to attain remission at least six months before planning conception. Serological test for anti Ro/LA antibody should be done in pregnancy lupus which is a marker to assess the risk of neonatal lupus and risk of increased maternal morbidity.

Treatment of lupus erythematosus includes general measures in the form of strict photo protection. Patients should be advised to conduct their activities early in the morning or late in the evening to avoid sun exposure. Basic change in lifestyle and habits like wearing full sleeve clothes which are tightly knit, use of broad brim hats, covering face with dupatta when going out in the sun are some measures which can go a long way in improving the quality of life of the patient. A good physical sunscreen with an adequate sun protection factor should also be advised. The sunscreen has to be applied on all the photo exposed parts at regular intervals of 2 to 3 hours starting from around 8:00 a.m. in the morning up to 3 p.m.

in the evening. Topical therapy includes the use of low to mid potency topical steroids. Calcineurin inhibitors like tacrolimus can be used as a useful adjunct and as a steroid sparing topical agent.

Oral therapy includes the use of oral corticosteroids which should be used judiciously and only when indicated specially to control acute disease flares, to tide over systemic involvement in the form of nephritis, vasculitis, or for neuropsychiatric involvement. Hydroxychloroquine (HCQ) besides acting as an oral photoprotective agent, also helps to decrease the risk of neonatal morbidity and adverse fetal outcomes like prematurity and growth retardation of the fetus. Hydroxychloroquine is considered safe in pregnancy and lactation. Azathioprine is another agent which can be used orally in case treatment with topical agents, corticosteroids and hydroxychloroquine is insufficient. Out of all the immunosuppressants, azathioprine is the agent of choice to be used in pregnant females due to its relatively better safety profile. Some recent studies have suggested a slightly increased risk of congenital heart disease in fetuses where the mother was on azathioprine during pregnancy. Thus risk benefit ratio should always be assessed before starting any immunosuppressive during pregnancy.

Antiphospholipid antibody syndrome (APLAS)

Antiphospholipid antibody syndrome can be seen in pregnant females in isolation or in association with autoimmune connective tissue disorders like lupus erythematosus, dermatomyositis, systemic sclerosis etc.

Pregnant females suffering from antiphospholipid antibody syndrome can present with thrombotic episodes, recurrent miscarriages and stillbirth. Serological tests in these patients often show positive antiphospholipid antibodies. They may also show a false positive VDRL test.

Once antiphospholipid antibody syndrome is diagnosed and there is no previous history of bad obstetric outcomes or thrombotic episodes; such patients should be started on low dose aspirin therapy. Patients who have a history of recurrent abortions or thrombosis should be started on combination therapy of low dose aspirin and low molecular weight heparin. Warfarin which is an oral drug used in the management of thrombosis should not be used in pregnant females due to its side effects. Hydroxychloroquine can also be added in such cases of antiphospholipid antibody syndrome especially if associated with cutaneous rash because of the known antithrombotic effect of hydroxychloroquine.

Systemic Sclerosis (SS)

Systemic sclerosis is a chronic autoimmune connective tissue disease characterized by progressive tightening and binding down of the skin associated with raynaud's phenomenon and systemic involvement mainly involving the respiratory, gastrointestinal and renal system.

Clinical presentation

Systemic sclerosis can be broadly categorized into three stages. The disease initially starts as the oedematous phase in which the patient often complains of tightening of ring on the fingers due to the edema and puffiness of fingers. The skin may also appear to be oedematous and shiny. This is followed by the second phase which is known as the induration phase in which the skin appears tight and indurated. In the later stages induration can increase and the skin may become bound down and tightly adherent to the underlying tissues. The skin changes may also be accompanied by pigmentary changes. The third and last phase is the atrophic phase which is characterized by generalized atrophy of the skin. Vascular manifestations include digital ulcerations and Raynaud's phenomenon.

Systemic Sclerosis and Pregnancy

Limited systemic sclerosis has a better prognosis in pregnant females than generalized systemic sclerosis. As far as the effect of pregnancy on systemic sclerosis is concerned; the course of systemic sclerosis is usually not greatly affected by pregnancy. The patients of systemic sclerosis may have an overall decreased fertility. Late age of onset of SS may be a reason because of which the data assessing the association of systemic sclerosis with pregnancy is inadequate. In fact some studies depicted decreased risk of systemic sclerosis in women who attained pregnancy compared with those who never got pregnant. Some other studies showed that the average longevity of the SS patients who gave childbirth was more as compared to those females who never conceived. Skin tightening and Raynaud's phenomenon usually improves during pregnancy. As a general rule whenever planning for conception, the disease activity of systemic sclerosis should ideally have been stabilized to ensure an uneventful pregnancy and childbirth. Adverse fetal outcomes have been reported in cases of systemic scleroderma especially when the disease is in active state; these include premature birth, spontaneous abortions and small for gestation babies. Cases of SS who have a significant risk of complications during pregnancy include the cases where the disease onset has been less than four years, diffuse type of systemic sclerosis, rapidly progressive disease and positive anti topoisomerase antibody. Pulmonary involvement is the most common cause of maternal morbidity followed by scleroderma renal crisis.

Management

All cases of systemic sclerosis should be counseled about the 'high risk' nature of pregnancy. Systemic sclerosis should be stabilized before planning for conception. Cases of systemic sclerosis who have aggressive disease, diffuse involvement and evidence of organ involvement should be counseled to delay planning pregnancy until the disease is brought under control. Most cases of systemic sclerosis improve during the pregnancy and thus may not need any active intervention other than a watchful approach to monitor fetal growth and identify any signs of fetal distress. Patients with limited skin involvement may be treated with moisturizers and topical steroids or calcineurin inhibitors like tacrolimus for skin complaints. In case of inadequate response to topical medications and the presence of widespread skin involvement narrow band UVB light can be administered. In cases of rapidly progressive disease and non-responders, a short course of oral corticosteroids can be added. In patients who require higher doses of corticosteroids, the use of a steroid sparing agent like azathioprine can be considered in consultation with the obstetrician and neonatologist.

Dermatomyositis(DM)

The exact etiology of dermatomyositis is not known, however there is a strong association of dermatomyositis with internal malignancies, drugs and pregnancy. The disease has a female predisposition. It is broadly of two types: the childhood type and adult type dermatomyositis.

Clinical Presentation

It is an autoimmune connective tissue disorder which involves the skin with or without the involvement of the musculoskeletal system. Skin lesions consist of reddish to violaceous rash involving the eyelids, cheeks and forehead often associated with edema and is known as **heliotrope rash**. Rash of a similar morphology when it appears on the neck and upper trunk is known as the **shawl sign**. Similar red and violaceous erythema may also be seen on the anterolateral surfaces of the thighs and extensor aspect of fingers known as **holster sign and gottron's sign** respectively. Pink to violaceous rounded papules present on the the interphalangeal joints of the hands are pathognomonic of dermatomyositis and are known as **gottron's papule**s. In severe cases, extension of the rash can give rise to an erythrodermic picture. Muscle involvement may manifest in the form of proximal muscle weakness where the patient complains of difficulty in standing from squatting position or difficulty in combing the hair. Lung involvement may also be seen and usually manifests in the form of parenchymal lung disease.

Dermatomyositis and pregnancy

Due to the late onset of dermatomyositis in adults usually after 40 years of age; dermatomyositis is not very common during pregnancy. Available data suggests that dermatomyositis improves during the pregnancy and can flare up again after delivery. TIF1-Gamma antibody has been associated with pregnancy induced dermatomyositis.

Dermatomyositis may be associated with adverse outcomes in pregnancy which includes increased incidence of abortion, prematurity and fetal growth retardation especially in those where the disease activity is not controlled before planning conception. Bad prognostic factors include active and severe disease during pregnancy, disease exacerbations happening during pregnancy and pregnancy induced dermatomyositis.

Management

Laboratory investigations may reveal elevated creatinine phosphokinase and aldolase levels except in the amyopathic dermatomyositis.

Management of dermatomyositis in pregnancy includes general photo protective measures. Use of sunscreens preferably physical, containing zinc oxide or titanium dioxide should be advised. For mild disease, topical therapy in the form of topical corticosteroids and calcineurin inhibitors like tacrolimus are used. For a more widespread disease, oral hydroxychloroquine can be added. In case the disease is not controlled with these drugs or if there is systemic involvement in the form of muscle or lung involvement; oral corticosteroids can be administered. Oral corticosteroids should be used judiciously to control the acute disease and later on steroid sparing agents like azathioprine can be used as a maintenance therapy. IVIG is another option which can be used to treat refractory cutaneous disease for muscle and lung involvement in dermatomyositis.

References

1. Griffith, C. E.M., & Baker, J. (Eds.). (2016). Rook's Textbook of Dermatology (9th ed., Vol. 3). Willey Blackwell.

2. Ingber, A. (2008). Obstetric Dermatology: A Practical Guide. Springer.

3. Tyler, K. H. (Ed.). (2020). Cutaneous Disorders of Pregnancy. Springer International Publishing.

4. Marder W, Littlejohn EA, Somers EC. Pregnancy and autoimmune connective tissue diseases. Best Pract Res Clin Rheumatol. 2016 Feb;30(1):63-80. doi: 10.1016/j.berh.2016.05.002. Epub 2016 Jun 25. Erratum in: Best Pract Res Clin Rheumatol. 2020 Dec;34(6):101490. PMID: 27421217; PMCID: PMC4947513.

5. Braunstein I, Werth V. Treatment of dermatologic connective tissue disease and autoimmune blistering disorders in pregnancy. Dermatol Ther. 2013;26(4):354–63.

6. Chen JS, Roberts CL, Simpson JM, March LM. Pregnancy outcomes in women with rare autoimmune diseases. Arthrit Rheumatol. 2015;67(12):3314–23.

7. Tedeschi SK, Massarotti E, Guan H, Fine A, Bermas BL, Costenbader KH. Specific systemic lupus erythematosus disease manifestations in the six months prior to conception are associated with similar disease manifestations during pregnancy. Lupus. 2015;24(12):1283–92.

8. Lateef A, Petri M. Managing lupus patients during pregnancy. Best Pract Res Clin Rheumatol. 2013;27(3):435–47.

9. Leroux M, Desveaux C, Parcevaux M, Julliac B, Gouyon J-B, Dallay D, et al. Impact of hydroxychloroquine on preterm delivery and intrauterine growth restriction in pregnant women with systemic lupus erythematosus: a descriptive cohort study. Lupus. 2015;24(13):1384–91.

10. Brucato A, Cimaz R, Caporali R, Ramoni V, Buyon J. Pregnancy outcomes in patients with autoimmune diseases and anti-Ro/SSA antibodies. Clin Rev Allergy Immunol. 2011;40(1):27-41. doi:10.1007/s12016-009-8190-6

11. Arese, Veronica & Murabito, Pierangela & Ribero, Simone & Panzone, Michele & Tonella, Luca & Fierro, Maria & Papini, Manuela & Quaglino, Pietro. (2019). Autoimmune connective tissue diseases and pregnancy. Giornale Italiano di Dermatologiae Venereologia. 154. 10.23736/S0392-0488.18.06252-1.

12. Rueda de Leon Aguirre A, Ramirez Calvo JA, Rodriguez Reyna TS. Comprehensive approach to systemic sclerosis patients during pregnancy. Reumatol Clin. 2015;11:99-107.

13. LidarM, Langevitz P. Pregnancy issues in scleroderma. Autoimmun Rev. 2012;11:A515-A519.

14. Clark KE, Etomi O, Ong VH. Systemic sclerosis in pregnancy. Obstet Med. 2020;13(3):105-111.

   doi:10.1177/1753495X19878042

15. Rao VK. Fertility and pregnancy in systemic sclerosis and other autoimmune rheumatic diseases. Indian J Rheumatol 2016;11, Suppl S2:150-5

16. Missumi LS, Souza FH, Andrade JQ, et al. Pregnancy outcomes in dermatomyositis and polymyositis patients. Rev Bras Reumatol. 2015;55:95-102.

17. Linardaki G, Cherouvim E, Goni G, et al. Intravenous immunoglobulin treatment for pregnancy-associated dermatomyositis. Rheumatol Int. 2011;31:113-115.

18. Oya K, Inoue S, Saito A, Nakamura Y, Ishitsuka Y, Fujisawa Y, et al. Pregnancy triggers the onset of anti-transcriptional intermediary factor 1γ antibody-positive dermatomyositis: a case series. Rheumatology. 2019.

Chapter 10

Pemphigus In Pregnancy

Pemphigus Vulgaris (PV)

It is an autoimmune vesiculobullous disease affecting the skin and the mucous membrane. It is characterized by an intra-epidermal level of split on histopathology. It is seen during the fifth and 6th decade of life, however in the Indian population it tends to appear a decade earlier.

Etiopathogenesis

It is an autoimmune disease characterized by the production of IgG autoantibodies directed against the transmembrane molecules known as the desmogleins, specifically desmoglein 1 and 3. Direct immunofluorescence studies have revealed intercellular deposition of immune reactants within the epidermis.

Clinical presentation

It presents in the form of skin and mucosal lesions. Skin lesions are in the form of flaccid vesicles and bullae which show peripheral extension and heal without scarring. **Nikolsky's sign and bulla spread sign** is positive in these cases. Usually the disease starts with lesions in the oral mucosa; in fact some patients may present with oral erosions only. The mucosal sites of involvement include the oral cavity and less commonly the nasal, ocular and genital mucosa. Skin involvement is predominantly seen on the scalp, face, upper trunk, axilla, groins and infra mammary areas but may later spread to involve the whole of the body.

Differential diagnosis

Pemphigus vulgaris in pregnancy should be differentiated from pemphigoid gestationis which is another autoimmune bullous disease with similar presentation. Unlike pemphigoid gestationis, PV usually presents with significant lesions involving the mucosae and flaccid blisters on the skin which rupture easily. Scaring and millia formation which occurs commonly in pemphigoid gestationis is not seen in pemphigus vulgaris. Further, skin biopsy and immunofluorescence studies can be done to differentiate PV from Pemphigoid gestationis.

Histopathology

Skin biopsy taken of the blister reveals the presence of an intra epidermal split with presence of multiple acantholytic cells within the blister cavity. The basal epidermal cells are attached to the underlying basement membrane but are separated from each other and the supra basal cells giving a characteristic **'Row of tombstone appearance'**. Direct immunofluorescence studies show deposition of IgG and C3 in the intraepidermal region in a **'fishnet'** pattern. Indirect immunofluorescence study is positive in more than 90% of the patients and correlates with the disease activity.

Pemphigus and pregnancy

Overall the course of pemphigus is not influenced by pregnancy; however PV may appear for the first time during pregnancy or pre existing lesions may get aggravated during the first or second trimester of pregnancy. Similar disease flares have been reported with the use of oral contraceptive pills underlining the role of hormones in aggravation of pemphigus. The disease activity of PV shows improvement during the third trimester of pregnancy which has been attributed to the production of endogenous steroids by the placenta in the later stages of pregnancy. After pregnancy the disease is seen to continue in its usual fashion characterized by remissions and exaggerations. Pregnancy should ideally not be planned unless the disease has stabilized and lesions have gone into remission and the antibody levels are at a low level. Adverse outcomes in the fetus have been reported when the maternal disease was poorly controlled and the antibody titres in the maternal serum were found to be high. This can be attributed to the severity of disease itself and the adverse effects of medications often used in high doses which are needed to control the disease activity of PV during the course of pregnancy.

In PV vertical transmission of IgG autoantibodies may lead to involvement of the neonatal skin and mucosa known as **neonatal pemphigus**. Fortunately neonatal pemphigus is often self limiting and the pathogenic autoantibodies usually get depleted from the fetal circulation within 2 to 3 weeks after which the cutaneous and mucosal involvement may settle down on its own. This severity of skin disease in the mother does not correspond with the increased incidence of neonatal pemphigus per se. Whether pemphigus vulgaris in pregnancy is associated with bad fetal outcome or not is debatable.

Pemphigus Foliaceus (PF)

PF is a variant of pemphigus group of disorders characterized by very fragile and superficial vesicles which rupture on their own and are distributed in a seborrheic distribution. These blisters often heel with thin corn flakes like brownish crust. Oral lesions are often mild or absent. In histopathology the blisters are situated at the level of the sub corneum. The disease usually has a chronic and indolent course.

Pemphigus foliaceus and pregnancy

Unlike PV, PF in the mothers does not predispose the neonate to develop the disease. Most neonates who are born to mothers suffering from PF are free of any cutaneous lesions during birth. The absence of cutaneous disease in neonates has been attributed to low titres of autoantibodies in the fetal circulation and the role of placenta in acting as a filter to prevent the passage of autoantibodies causing PF into the fetal circulation. Some studies have highlighted the role of different desmogleins involved as compared to PV. Superficial epidermis of the fetus has high expression of desmoglein 3 which explains the lack of cutaneous lesions in the fetus of the mother suffering from PF.

Management of Pemphigus

Corticosteroids including the topical and oral corticosteroids are the front runners in drug therapy of pemphigus during pregnancy. In mild and localized cases that treatment should start with the use of topical steroids or calcineurin inhibitors. Intralesional steroid therapy with the use of injection triamcinolone 10 mg per ml can be used in isolated and recalcitrant lesions of oral pemphigus. Secondary infections should be treated with oral or parenteral antibiotics. In cases where additional therapy is required, oral corticosteroids preferably prednisolone should be used for the initial control of the disease. Azathioprine has been used as a second line drug in cases where adequate response has not been achieved with the use of corticosteroids. However in such cases it should be started after completion of the first trimester of pregnancy keeping in view the risk benefit ratio of the drug. IVIG and plasmapheresis have also been tried in selected cases. Other drugs which have been tried in pregnancy include oral dapsone and rituximab.

References

1. Griffith, C. E.M., & Baker, J. (Eds.). (2016). Rook's Textbook of Dermatology (9th ed., Vol. 3). Willey Blackwell.

2. Ingber, A. (2008). Obstetric Dermatology: A Practical Guide. Springer.

3. Tyler, K. H. (Ed.). (2020). Cutaneous Disorders of Pregnancy. Springer International Publishing.

4. Fagundes PPS, Santi CG, Maruta CW, Miyamoto D, Aoki V. Autoimmune bullous diseases in pregnancy: clinical and epidemiological characteristics and therapeutic approach. An Bras Dermatol. 2021;96(5):581-590.

   doi:10.1016/j.abd.2020.10.007

5. Patsatsi A, Marinovic B, Murrell D. Autoimmune bullous diseases during pregnancy: Solving common and uncommon issues. Int J Womens Dermatol. 2019;5(3):166-170. Published 2019 Jan 24. doi:10.1016/j.ijwd.2019.01.003

6. Lin L, Zeng X, Chen Q. Pemphigus and pregnancy. Analysis and summary of case reports over 49 years. Saudi Med J. 2015;36(9):1033-1038. doi:10.15537/smj.2015.9.12270

7. KardosM, Levine D, Gurcan HM, et al. Pemphigus vulgaris in pregnancy: Analysis of current data on the management and outcomes. Obstet Gynecol Surv. 2009;64:739-749.

8. Ahmed AR, Gurcan HM. Use of intravenous immunoglobulin therapy during pregnancy in patients with pemphigus vulgaris. J Eur Acad Dermatol Venereol. 2011;25:1073-1079.

9. Daneshpazhooh M, Chams-Davatchi C, Valikhani M, Aghabagheri A, Mortazavizadeh SM, Barzegari M, Akhyani M, Hallaji Z, Esmaili N, Ghodsi S Z. Pemphigus and pregnancy: A 23-year experience. Indian J Dermatol Venereol Leprol 2011;77:534

10. M. Kokolios, F. Lamprou, D. Stylianidou, D. Sotiriadis, A. Patsatsi, New onset pemphigus foliaceus during pregnancy: A rare case International Journal of Women's Dermatology, Volume 4, Issue 2, 2018

Chapter 11

Skin Infections Associated With Pregnancy

Introduction

Skin infections occurring during pregnancy include viral, fungal, bacterial, spirochetal, protozoal and parasitic infections. Vaginitis specially candidal vulvovaginitis is the most commonly found skin infection associated with pregnancy. The increased level of hormones especially estrogen during pregnancy causes a shift of adaptive immune response towards the Th2 mediated pathway which results in impairment of cell mediated immunity. This makes pregnancy a state of relative immunosuppression and makes the female body more susceptible to a variety of infections. The hormonal and immunological alterations which take place during pregnancy have a significant effect on the presentation and natural course of these infections. Some infectious diseases can have adverse maternal and fetal outcomes if acquired during pregnancy. The drug therapy required to treat these infections has to be curated very carefully in order to avoid any harmful effects of medications to the mother and the fetus. Discussion regarding every infection which occurs during pregnancy is beyond the scope of this book. However infections which carry a significant importance in relation to pregnancy shall be discussed in this chapter.

Vulvovaginal candidiasis

Candida is a normal commensal yeast present in the vaginal flora in around 25% of the sexually active females. As discussed already it is one of the most common infections seen in pregnancy perhaps because of the high levels of estrogen leading to an overproduction of vaginal glycogen and suppression of the cell mediated immune response in pregnancy. Candidal vaginitis is often more severe and more symptomatic during pregnancy as compared to that in non pregnant females. It is more common during the second and third trimester of pregnancy. The patients usually complain of intense itching, burning sensation and thick curdy white vaginal discharge. Microscopic examination of the vaginal discharge using 10% potassium hydroxide to demonstrate fungal elements can confirm the diagnosis of candidiasis. Some patients may also complain of burning maturation. Recent studies have suggested an increased risk of premature rupture of membrane, preterm labor and congenital candidiasis. Congenital candidiasis can occur due to intrauterine spread of the Candidal infection to the fetus. Candidiasis in the neonate can also develop during delivery as a result of ascending infection through the birth canal. The neonate may present with candidiasis involving the oral mucosa, angle of the mouth (perleche) or as peri anal trush. Treatment of vulvovaginal candidiasis in pregnancy is done with topical antifungals or vaginal pessary to avoid systemic exposure of drugs. The aim of therapy is to provide symptomatic relief and to prevent development of pregnancy related complications caused by vaginal candidiasis. Oral fluconazole is better avoided especially at high doses because of the reports of congenital abnormalities seen due to the use of oral fluconazole in some studies especially during the first trimester.

Bacterial vaginosis

It is another common type of vaginal infection seen in both pregnant and non pregnant females. It is seen due to the disturbance of normal vaginal flora from predominance of healthy hydrogen peroxide producing lactobacilli to increase in anaerobic bacteria like gardnerella, mobiluncus, and mycoplasma species. Clinical diagnosis can be made with the help of Amsel's criteria.

Figure 5

AMSEL'S CRITERIA

- pH of more than 4.5
- Fishy or amine order on instilling a drop of potassium hydroxide on vaginal discharge (Whiff's Test)
- Presence of clue cells which are vaginal epithelial cells coated with bacilli on the borders
- Presence of a homogenous vaginal discharge

There have been reports of adverse fetal outcomes associated with bacterial vaginosis however there is no concrete data to suggest that treatment of bacterial vaginosis during pregnancy can prevent such complications.

Treatment consists of topical clindamycin cream to be applied for seven consecutive nights. It is the only treatment which is safe to be used during the first trimester. Oral metronidazole in the dose of 400 mg thrice daily can be used in the second and third trimester for a period of 1 week. A combination of metronidazole and erythromycin has shown to be more efficacious in preventing preterm births. Oral clindamycin has also been used and found to be largely safe in pregnancy. There is no evidence however that treatment of bacterial vaginosis infection can prevent adverse pregnancy outcomes.

Trichomonal vaginitis

It is another common type of vaginal infection caused by a protozoa known as *trichomonas vaginalis*. The infection is often asymptomatic, however some patients may complain of itching, burning, and redness of the vulvovaginal region with or without dysuria. On clinical examination the vaginal wall and cervix appear intense red in color also known as **strawberry cervix**. The vaginal discharge is characteristically greenish in color and often gives an ammoniacal or fishy smell. A useful bedside test is the preparation of a saline mount of the vaginal discharge which on microscopic examination can reveal the trichomonas virginialis as a motile, ovoid shaped flagellated organism with a characteristic motility.

Trichomonas infection in pregnancy especially during the second trimester has been associated with adverse fetal outcomes in the form of preterm birth, intrauterine growth retardation and premature rupture of membranes. Prophylactic screening and treatment of asymptomatic cases is not recommended and not known to decrease the risk of bad obstetric outcome in pregnancy. Symptomatic cases can be treated with oral metronidazole 400 mg thrice a day for 7 days during the second or third trimester. However, there is no evidence that treatment of trichomonas infection can prevent adverse outcomes in pregnancy.

Herpes zoster and chickenpox infection in pregnancy

Varicella zoster virus (VZV) infection in pregnancy can present in a number of ways depending upon the immune status of the mother and the timing of acquiring infection during the course of pregnancy.

1. Herpes zoster infection in pregnancy

Herpes zoster (HZ) also known as *shingles* is a viral infection caused by reactivation of varicella zoster virus from the dermatomal ganglion. In a usual case of herpes zoster, the viral spread is usually segmental or dermatomal and presence of virus in the circulation is not seen except in the cases of disseminated herpes zoster. Because of the absence of viremia, the transplacental spread from the mother to the child is highly unlikely. As a general rule, an episode of herpes zoster does not translate into severe adverse outcomes for the mother or the fetus. Severe forms of herpes zoster like disseminated, multi dermatomal, HZ ophthalmicus and HZ oticus should be treated with parenteral acyclovir.

2. Varicella/Chickenpox in pregnancy

Varicella also known as *chickenpox* is a primary infection caused by VZV in a previously non exposed pregnant female. Chickenpox tends to have a more severe outcome in pregnancy as compared to herpes zoster especially during the third trimester of pregnancy in terms of maternal morbidity. The risk of developing systemic involvement in chickenpox associated with pregnancy is quite high and is associated with a high mortality rate. The most common systemic complication seen with chickenpox in pregnancy is varicella pneumonia followed by hepatitis and CNS involvement. Fetal prognosis in most of the cases of chickenpox in pregnancy remains good. Although fetoplacental transmission of VZV is seen in one out of 4 cases of maternal chickenpox, congenital varicella syndrome develops in only one to two percent of these cases. In cases who develop chickenpox during pregnancy, fetal and maternal monitoring should be done. Termination of pregnancy is not usually indicated unless the fetal scans depict any serious anomalies in the fetus. The risk of spontaneous abortion with chicken pox in pregnancy is seen to be around 8%.

Management

In cases of a recent onset rash less than 72 hours in duration oral acyclovir in the dose of 800 mg 5 times a day should be started. It is seen to reduce both maternal and fetal morbidity. In case of chickenpox associated with complications like pneumonia, hepatitis or CNS symptoms; in cases where the lesions are persisting or hemorrhagic, intravenous acyclovir in the dose of 10mg per kg body weight 8 hourly should be initiated. Acyclovir and valacyclovir are considered to be safe for use in pregnancy and are not known to cause significant fetal malformations.

3. Congenital varicella syndrome

Congenital varicella syndrome is a condition seen in newborns born to mothers who had suffered an episode of chickenpox during pregnancy leading to the fetoplacental spread of virus in-utero. The neonate usually presents with dermatomal lesions and ulcerations resembling that of herpes zoster along with scarring and contracture formation. The risk of developing congenital varicella syndrome is more if the infection is acquired before 20 weeks of gestation; it is maximum during the second trimester of pregnancy. Congenital varicella syndrome is a serious condition and carries a high mortality risk of 30% or more. Ocular involvement in the form of microphthalmia, chorioretinitis and cataract can be seen in more than 50% of the cases. Musculoskeletal abnormalities in the form of limb hypoplasia and abnormalities of digits can be seen in around 80% of the cases. Central nervous system can also be involved and some neonates may present with microcephaly. Other complications include reduced birth weight and growth retardation. Other organs including the cardiovascular system and the gastrointestinal system may also be involved, although less commonly.

The neonates should be treated aggressively with intravenous acyclovir in order to prevent progression of congenital varicella syndrome.

4. Infantile herpes zoster

Herpes zoster may develop in an infant during the first year of his life when the mother acquires chicken pox during the second or third trimester of pregnancy. Herpes zoster during the first year of life usually develops due to the poorly developed cellular immune response of the infant. The course of disease is usually self limiting and skin lesions usually resolve within 2 weeks. In case herpes zoster lesions are disseminated or multi-dermatomal; involve the eyes or face; or there is associated immunosuppression, in such cases active treatment with intravenous acyclovir is required.

5. Chicken pox in a neonate

Chicken pox can develop in a newborn if the mother acquires infection of VZV during the period of delivery. The highest risk of developing chicken pox in the neonate is when the mother acquires infection within a week before delivery to a week after it. The risk of developing neonatal varicella in such cases is very high, often up to 50% in some cases. The chicken pox infection in neonates usually manifests within the second week of birth in most cases. This is believed to happen because the cellular immune response of the neonate is not well developed during this period as the protective maternal antibodies transferred from the mother to the fetus are not adequate. The viral infection usually spreads from the mother to the fetus through placental route or through droplet mode or as an ascending infection through the birth canal during delivery. Neonatal chickenpox can present itself in the form of a generalized eruption sometimes with the presence of hemorrhagic blisters. The disease course can be severe with involvement of multiple organ systems manifesting in the form of pneumonia, encephalitis, hepatitis, myocarditis, orchitis and small vessel vasculitis. The mortality rate is often very high ranging from 20 to 30%. However timely therapy in the form of intravenous acyclovir can bring down the mortality rate to around 10%. Prophylactic measures in case the mother develops chickenpox one week before delivery include postponement of elective delivery if possible, administration of VZV immunoglobulin, isolation of mother from child after delivery and observation of the neonate for 2 weeks after birth. The mother should be started on acyclovir as soon as varicella is diagnosed in order to reduce viral shedding and decrease the chances of transmission to the fetus. If the neonate has developed lesions of chickenpox intravenous acyclovir therapy should be started immediately in the dose of 10 to 20 mg per kg body weight 8 hourly for 1 to 2 weeks.

Genital warts in pregnancy

Genital warts also known as **condyloma acuminata** is a type of viral infection caused by human papillomavirus mainly of types 6, 11, 16 and 18. Type 6 and 11 have low oncogenic risk and are usually associated with genital warts whereas type 16 and 18 are more commonly associated with genital dysplasias, especially cervical cancers. Genital warts usually present as papillated and cauliflower-like vegetating fleshy lesions which are pale or pink coloured involving the female genital area like the vulva, clitoris, vaginal canal and cervix. Pregnancy has a positive effect on the growth of genital warts which are seen to become larger in size during the course of pregnancy especially around 12 to 14 weeks of gestation. It is believed to be caused due to the impaired cell mediated immunity and increased vascularity of the genital area during pregnancy which favors the growth and proliferation of human papilloma virus. As a result of this, the genital warts become more fleshy and bulky as well as more friable during pregnancy. In some cases, the warts can enlarge too much in size causing obstruction of the external genital tract making vaginal delivery difficult. In such cases cesarean delivery has to be undertaken. Cesarean delivery is not otherwise mandated in cases of condyloma acuminata except in case of obstruction of the birth canal or extensive bleeding from the warts or premature rupture of membranes. Transmission of human papillomavirus infection can occur from mother to the child during delivery which can result in development of lesions in the neonate involving the anogenital area, oral cavity and the conjunctiva. Transmission of infection during the intranatal period has also been described to cause laryngeal papilloma in some neonates. However there is no evidence to suggest that cesarean delivery can prevent the occurrence of laryngeal papillomatosis in the fetus. Fetal complications in the form of placental abnormalities and preterm delivery have been reported in infections caused by HPV 16 and 18.

Preventive measures can include the administration of human papillomavirus vaccines which include bivalent, quadrivalent and nonavalent HPV vaccines designed for use in women of reproductive age for prevention of future HPV infections. However they are not to be used during pregnancy.

Management

Treatment of genital warts in pregnancy includes both medical and surgical modalities. Surgical modalities which are considered safe during pregnancy include electro-cauterization, cryotherapy, scalpel excision and carbon dioxide laser ablation. Cryotherapy is considered to be the preferred surgical modality in pregnancy. Medical treatments include chemical cauterization with trichloroacetic acid (75 to 100 percent) however it is less effective in thicker religions as compared to surgical modalities. Other medical treatments which have been used in genital warts in non pregnant patients include podophyllotoxin, salicylic acid, imiquimod and sinecatechin. However, these agents are better avoided during pregnancy because of the lack of safety data in pregnancy.

Herpes simplex infection in pregnancy

Herpes viruses are a group of double stranded DNA viruses. Herpes simplex virus (HSV) is a member of the herpes virus family and is transmitted through direct mucosal contact during the primary infection. HSV infection is one of the most common sexually transmitted infections worldwide. HSV is of two types HSV1 and HSV2. HSV type 1 is known to cause oral gingivostomatitis and ocular infections in the form of keratoconjunctivitis. Genital herpes simplex infection can be caused by both HSV1 and HSV2. The incubation period may vary from two days to 2 weeks. HSV infection during pregnancy does not pose a serious risk for maternal health, however neonatal infection of herpes simplex can have serious consequences for the newborn. Genital herpes in the mother during the primary episode presents with painful ulcerations of the genitalia along with systemic features in the form of fever, urinary tract complaints, lymphadenopathy and dysuria. Recurrent genital herpes infection is caused by intermittent reactivation of the herpes virus from the neuronal ganglia leading to grouped vesicles and erosions in the genitalia often in the absence of systemic features. Recurrent genital herpes has a shorter incubation period and usually subsides without scarring and in a shorter span of time as compared to primary episode of herpes. Neonatal transmission of herpes can occur even in the absence of a clinically apparent maternal infection due to the asymptomatic viral shedding through the maternal reproductive tract. Maternal herpes infection during pregnancy is a part of the congenital TORCH complex of infections and may present with serious complications to the neonate in the form of severe cutaneous lesions and systemic findings including neurological abnormalities. The incidence of neonatal herpes simplex infection is maximum when the infection is acquired by the mother around the time of delivery. The maximum risk of developing neonatal herpes simplex virus infection is when the mother acquires genital herpes infection for the first time during pregnancy. Patients who have an active herpes infection during the time of delivery should undergo cesarean section in order to decrease the chances of transmission to the neonate during childbirth. The fetal prognosis is good when the neonatal infection is localized to the skin. In cases of widespread skin infection along with systemic involvement the mortality is high and if the neonate survives the chances of developing disability and sequelae is quite common .

In case a pregnant woman presents with doubtful lesions suggestive of a possible herpes simplex infection of the genitalia, viral culture should be done. In case the female complaints of symptoms suggestive of herpes simplex infection of the genitalia without the presence of clinical lesions, serological tests to detect herpes virus antibodies should be done. HSV DNA PCR test is usually the most sensitive test to detect the presence of herpes simplex virus in genital secretions, however it is often available in specialized centers only.

Management

Treatment of genital herpes simplex virus infection in pregnancy is done using oral antivirals like acyclovir, famciclovir and valacyclovir. All of these drugs are pregnancy category B drugs however acyclovir is usually preferred due to the considerable history of use and safety data in pregnancy. For the primary episode of genital herpes in pregnancy acyclovir is given at a dose of 400 mg 3 times a day for 7 to 10 days. In cases of recurrent genital herpes, acyclovir is given at a dose of 400 mg 3 times a day or 800 mg twice daily for 5 days. In case of repeated episodes of herpes simplex treated with suppressive therapy of acyclovir, a dose of 400 mg thrice daily is usually started at 36 weeks and continued until delivery.

Pityriasis rosea in pregnancy

Etiopathogenesis

PR has been found to be associated with infection of human herpesvirus 6 and 7. The increased incidence of pregnancy can be attributed to increased chances of acquiring HHV 6 and 7 infection due to pregnancy being a state of impaired cellular immunity.

Clinical presentation

Pityriasis rosea is a papulosquamous eruption associated with HHV 6 and HHV 7 virus infection presenting in young adults and characterized by sudden eruption of red scaly papules and plaques distributed along the truncal lines in a *'Christmas tree'* or an *'inverted fir tree'* appearance. Prodromal symptoms in the form of malaise, sore throat, arthralgias and fever can precede the eruption. The initial skin lesion before the generalized eruption can appear in the form of a large oval scaly plaque with the scales arranged in a collarette-like fashion known as **herald patch** or **mother patch**.

The prevalence of pregnancy is much higher than what is expected in non pregnant females of the same age. There have been reports of adverse fetal outcomes in infections acquired during pregnancy which include spontaneous abortions, stillbirths, premature delivery and neonatal hypotonia especially when the infection was acquired before 20 weeks of gestation. The adverse neonatal outcome has been associated with the transplacental spread of underlying HHV 6 and 7 infection during the first trimester. On the other hand many other studies did not find any significant fetal risks associated with PR in pregnancy. However it is worthwhile to screen the fetus for any congenital abnormality and fetal distress in females suffering from PR during pregnancy.

Management

PR in pregnancy does not require treatment in all the cases as the condition follows a self limiting course. In case of symptomatic lesions, topical steroids and emollients can be used. Most of the cases of PR show complete settlement of rash within 2 months of onset. Since PR acquired in the first trimester of pregnancy has been reported to be associated with adverse fetal outcome especially in cases of widespread rash persisting for a longer duration or rash associated with constitutional symptoms. It may be worthwhile to start such patients on oral acyclovir at a dose of 800 mg 5 times a day for 7 to 10 days which has shown to decrease the extent of rash and the time required in clearance of the eruption especially when the treatment is started within one week of onset of the rash. Oral acyclovir being a pregnancy category B drug can be instituted in selected cases considering the risk benefit analysis.

Human Immunodeficiency Virus (HIV) infection in pregnancy

HIV infection is a viral infection caused by RNA retrovirus. It usually stays in a state of latency for a long period often extending up to years before manifesting clinically as auto immune deficiency syndrome (AIDS). It presents in the form of clinical immunosuppression characterized by the frequent secondary infections like tuberculosis, weight loss, prolonged fever, diarrhea and generalized lymphadenopathy.

Increased blood volume and haemodilution seen in pregnancy can give a false low CD4 count value. Whether pregnancy has an effect on the course of HIV infection is unclear. Pregnant females suffering from HIV infection are reported to have unfavorable fetal outcomes in the form of spontaneous abortion, stillbirth, intrauterine growth retardation and preterm delivery. Mother-to-child transmission is seen most commonly during the period of labor and during breastfeeding. The risk of transmission of HIV infection from mother to child varies from around 15 to 45% in the absence of treatment. However if proper treatment is instituted the risk decreases to 5% or less.

In pregnant females who suffer from HIV infection, antiretroviral therapy (HAART) should be given in all the cases and continued throughout the period of pregnancy and delivery. ART has been shown to improve obstetric outcomes in pregnancy and reduce mother to child transmission. In case of a low viral load, the chances of transmission of infection to the child through vaginal delivery is very low hence the vaginal route of delivery can be undertaken. However if the viral load at the time of delivery is found to be high, the route of cesarean section should be undertaken for childbirth. Breastfeeding is usually continued in HIV positive females while continuing to take ART. Exclusive breastfeeding can be given for 6 months followed by introduction of top feed. If the mother has received less than 4 months of ART or has high viral load, the neonate can be given a short course of ART for 6 weeks consisting of once a day nevirapine and twice a day zidovudine. HIV positive infants should be given prophylaxis for pneumocystis infection with cotrimoxazole.

Syphilis in pregnancy

Syphilis is a sexually transmitted disease which can present in a variety of ways and is primarily divided into primary, secondary, latent and tertiary syphilis The clinical presentation of syphilis is not seen to be largely altered by pregnancy. Transmission from mother to child can occur at any time and during any stage of syphilis. The risk of transmission from mother to child depends on this spirochaetal load present in the maternal blood. Early syphilis consisting of primary and secondary stages of syphilis carry a higher risk of transmission from mother to child because of high spirochaetal load. On the other hand latent and tertiary syphilis have a less risk of transmission from mother to child due to the lowest spirochaetal count in the maternal blood. The most problematic complication of syphilis in pregnancy is the occurrence of congenital syphilis. The presentation of congenital syphilis depends on various factors like the gestation age at the time of infection, stage of maternal syphilis and the immunological status of the fetus. Syphilis in pregnancy can be associated with adverse fetal outcomes in the form of intrauterine growth retardation, hydrops fetalis (non-immune type), premature delivery, spontaneous abortion and stillbirth. Overall, it is seen that around ⅓ rd of pregnancies result in abortion or stillbirth, while 1/3rd fetuses develop congenital syphilis and another 1/3rd are born healthy. The diagnosis and treatment of syphilis in pregnancy remains more or less same as that of the non pregnant population. Non-treponemal and treponemal serological tests for syphilis are used to diagnose females with syphilis. Early treatment of syphilis in pregnancy is important as it helps to prevent fetal complications by instituting timely treatment. The treatment of choice of syphilis in pregnancy remains the same as the non pregnant population. In early cases of syphilis a total dose of 2.4 million units of benzathine penicillin is given as half dose on each buttock. In late syphilis, 2.4 million units are given as weekly doses for 3 weeks. Second line drugs like doxycycline and tetracycline are not to be used during pregnancy because of their teratogenicity.

Scabies in pregnancy

Pregnant females are at a greater risk of acquiring scabies infestation which is an infection caused by a mite known as *sarcoptes scabiei*. The possibility of a scabies infestation should always be considered in pregnant females presenting with an itchy skin condition.

Topical permethrin 5% remains the treatment of choice for scabies in pregnancy due to its proven safety and efficacy. Topical benzyl benzoate 25% can be used as a second line agent for the treatment of scabies in pregnancy. Topical sulfur is also considered to be safe in pregnancy however it is not easily available and the application is often messy and staining of clothes is often reported after application of topical sulfur preparation. Topical treatment should be repeated after a week to kill the ova and persistent mites. All the possible contacts should be advised to get treated to prevent cross infection. Topical treatment in the form of steroid antibiotic combination can be given for the excoriated and itchy lesions. First generation oral antihistamines can be given for itching and sleep disturbance caused by scabies.

Topical agents like Gamma benzene hexachloride and malathion should not be used in pregnancy due to their adverse effects. Oral ivermectin is also better avoided in pregnancy.

Leprosy in pregnancy

Leprosy is a chronic infectious disease caused by an acid fast bacillus known as the *mycobacterium leprae*. It is an intracellular bacillus the fate of which depends on the host cell mediated immunity to adequately contain the infection. Since pregnancy is a state of immune suppression characterized by a decrease in the cell mediated immunity, pregnancy can logically have deleterious effects on the course of leprosy. ENL in pregnancy is associated with early loss of neuronal function as compared to the routine cases of leprosy. Neuronal deterioration is much more rapid and more common in pregnant females having leprosy and neurological examination should be done at regular intervals to detect any nerve function impairment and in order to initiate early treatment of the same. Reaction states in leprosy are also more commonly seen in pregnant females as compared to the non pregnant population. There is also a theoretical possibility of increased drug resistance due to the impaired cellular immune response seen in pregnancy. In case a female is diagnosed with leprosy before conceiving, it is better to plan the pregnancy after the treatment course of leprosy has been completed and the patient is free of any reactions. Patients who are diagnosed to have leprosy in pregnancy should undergo treatment with multi drug therapy prescribed by WHO as in non pregnant cases of leprosy. Leprosy reactions in pregnancy should be treated with oral steroids in tapering doses, however the use of some medications like immunosuppressive agents is usually not recommended because of their teratogenic and other side effects.

References

1. Khan F, Mays RM, Brooks J, Tyring SK. Viral and sexually transmitted disease. In: Kroumpouzos G, ed. Text Atlas of Obstetric Dermatology. Philadelphia.

2. Puri K J, Madan A, Bajal K. Evaluation of causes of vaginal discharge in relation to pregnancy status. Indian J Dermatol Venereol Leprol 2003;69:129-130

3. Aguin TJ, Sobel JD. Vulvovaginal candidiasis in pregnancy. Curr Infect Dis Rep. 2015;17:462.

4. Fardiazar Z, Ronaci F, Torab R, Goldust M. Vulvovaginal candidiasis recurrence during pregnancy. Pak J Biol Sci. 2012;15:399-402.

5. Kumar N, Behera B, Sagiri SS, Pal K, Ray SS, Roy S. Bacterial vaginosis: Etiology and modalities of treatment-A brief note. J Pharm Bioallied Sci. 2011;3(4):496-503. doi:10.4103/0975-7406.90102

6. US Preventive Services Task Force. Screening for Bacterial Vaginosis in Pregnant Persons to Prevent Preterm Delivery: US Preventive Services Task Force Recommendation Statement. JAMA. 2020;323(13):1286–1292. doi:10.1001/jama.2020.2684

7. Cotch MF, Pastorek II JG, Nugent RP, et al. Trichomonas vaginalis associated with low birth weight and preterm delivery. The Vaginal Infections and Prematurity Study Group. Sex Transm Dis. 1997;24:353-360.

8. Lamont RF, Sobel JD, Carrington D, et al. Varicella-zoster virus (chickenpox) infection in pregnancy. BJOG. 2011;118(10):1155-1162.

doi:10.1111/j.1471-0528.2011.02983.x

9. Ghosh S, Chaudhuri S. Pregnancy and varicella infection: A resident's quest. Indian J Dermatol Venereol Leprol 2013;79:264-267

10. Wiwanitkit V. Chicken pox in pregnancy : An obstetric concern. Indian J Dermatol 2010;55:313-5

11. Dana A, Buchanan KM, Goss MA, et al. Pregnancy outcomes from the pregnancy registry of a human papillomavirus type 6/1116/18 vaccine. Obstet Gynecol. 2009;114:1170-1178.

12. Tenti P, Zappatore R, Migliora P, Spinillo A, Belloni C, Carnevali L. Perinatal transmission of human papillomavirus virus from pregnant with latent infections. Obstet Gynecol. 1999;93:475-479.

13. Silverberg MJ, Thorsen P, Lindeberg H, et al. Condyloma in pregnancy is strongly predictive of juvenile-onset recurrent respiratory papillomatosis. Obstet Gynecol. 2003;101:645-652.

14. Stephenson-Famy A, Gardella C. Herpes simplex virus infection during pregnancy. Obstet Gynecol Clin North Am. 2014:41601-41614.

15. Starface G, Selmin A, Zanardo V, De Santis M, Ercoli A, Scambia G. Herpes simplex virus infection in pregnancy. Infect Dis Obstet Gynecol. 2012;2012:385697.

doi:10.1155/2012/385697

16. Su CW, McKay B. Treatment of HSV infection in late pregnancy. Am Fam Physician. 2012;85:390-393.

17. Kimberlin DW. Neonatal herpes simplex infection. Clin Microbiol Rev. 2004;17:1-13.

18. Brown ZA, Wald A, Morrow RA, Selke S, Zeh J, Corey L. Effect of serologic status and cesarean delivery on transmission rates of herpes simplex virus from mother to infant. JAMA. 2003;289:203-209.

19. Loh TY, Cohen PR. Pityriasis rosea in pregnancy: report of a spousal occurrence and craniosynostosis in the healthy newborn. Dermatol Pract Concept. 2016;6(3):39-46. Published 2016 Jul 31. doi:10.5826/dpc.0603a08

20. Wenger-Oehn, L., Graier, T., Ambros- Rudolph, C., Müllegger, R., Bittighofer, C., Wolf, P. and Hofer, A. (2022), Pityriasis rosea in pregnancy: A case series and literature review. JDDG: Journal der Deutschen Dermatologischen Gesellschaft, 20: 953-959. https://doi.org/10.1111/ddg.14763

21. Irshad U, Mahdy H, Tonismae T. HIV In Pregnancy. [Updated 2022 Sep 20]. In: StatPearls [Internet]. Treasure Island (FL): StatPearls Publishing; 2022 Jan-. Available from: https://www.ncbi.nlm.nih.gov/books/NBK558972/

22. Wahab AA, Ali UK, Mohammad M, Md Monoto EM, Rahman MM. Syphilis in pregnancy. Pak J Med Sci. 2015;31(1):217-219. doi:10.12669/pjms.311.5932

23. Trinh T, Leal AF, Mello MB, et al. Syphilis management in pregnancy: a review of guideline recommendations from countries around the world. Sex Reprod Health Matters. 2019;27(1):69-82. doi:10.1080/26410397.2019.1691897

24. Patel VM, Lambert W C, Schwartz RA. Safety of topical medications for scabies and lice in pregnancy. Indian J Dermatol 2016;61:583-7

25. Ozturk Z, Tatliparmak A. Leprosy treatment during pregnancy and breastfeeding: A case report and brief review of literature. Dermatol Ther. 2017 Jan;30(1). doi: 10.1111/dth.12414. Epub 2016 Aug 23. PMID: 27549245.

Chapter 12

Diseases Affecting The Sebaceous Glands In Pregnancy

The hormonal changes which occur during the pregnancy are believed to cause an increase in the activity of sebaceous glands especially during the later half of pregnancy where the patients may complain of increased oiliness of skin and increased predisposition to develop acne.

Acne vulgaris in pregnancy

Acne vulgaris is a common disorder of the pilosebaceous unit characterized by development of a variety of lesions including comedones, inflammatory papules, pustules and nodulocystic lesions usually arising after the onset of puberty. The management of acne vulgaris in pregnancy can be a tricky situation for the clinician because some of the commonly used drugs for treatment of acne like oral isotretinoin are contraindicated to be used in pregnancy because of their teratogenic effects.

Etiopathogenesis

Acne vulgaris is believed to develop because of multiple contributory factors which include an increased sebaceous activity secondary to the surge in androgenic hormones seen during puberty as well as in pregnancy. The factors which contribute to the development of acne vulgaris include increased sebum production from the sebaceous glands, proliferation of *Propionibacterium acnes* within the follicle which triggers an inflammatory response and the role of follicular hyperkeratosis. The role of diet in acne is controversial and recent studies indicate that dietary changes have an insignificant effect on the course of acne.

Pregnancy is characterized by an increase in the level of hormones like estrogen, progesterone and hcg. These hormonal changes are believed to stimulate the activity of sebaceous glands. The impaired glucose tolerance and increased insulin levels seen in some females during pregnancy have also been associated with increased incidence of acne. Hyperinsulinemia has been associated with increase in the sebocyte activity through the growth hormone receptors present on the sebaceous cells.

Clinical presentation

The clinical presentation can be varied and the patients may present with a variety of lesions ranging from comedones which can be closed or open, inflammatory papules, pustules and nodulocystic regions. Most of the acne patients present with lesions on the face, however involvement of the upper chest, shoulders and back can also be seen.

The course of acne in pregnancy is variable ranging from improvement of acne in some cases and deterioration in others. Most of the acne exacerbations in pregnancy are seen during the third trimester when the sebaceous gland activity is at its peak. Some patients may complain of severe forms of acne during the postpartum period known as post gestational acne.

Differential diagnosis

Acne in pregnancy should be differentiated from other acneiform eruptions like perioral dermatitis, rosacea and steroid induced acneiform eruptions. Acne vulgaris can be differentiated from acneiform eruptions by the presence of comedonal lesions which are characteristic of acne vulgaris and the predominant facial distribution.

Management

The armament of treatment in acne during pregnancy is often restricted. Most clinicians follow a conservative approach to avoid any side effects to the fetus and since acne exacerbated during pregnancy is believed to subside after delivery, it is often justifiable as well. Conservative treatment in the form of topical antibiotics can be given especially during the first trimester of pregnancy. Systemic drugs which are safe like azithromycin can be considered in more severe forms of acne.

Topical azelaic acid which has anti-inflammatory and antimicrobial properties is safe for use in pregnancy being a FDA category B drug. It also has the advantage of improvement in acne induced pigmentation because of its property to inhibit tyrosinase.

Other safe options include topical antibiotic agents like erythromycin and clindamycin which are pregnancy category B preparations. They have antimicrobial properties against P. acnes.

Other topical preparations like benzoyl peroxide, salicylic acid and glycolic acid are pregnancy category C drugs and should either be avoided during pregnancy or the patient should be advised against using it on a larger surface area so as to prevent significant systemic absorption. Topical retinoids like tretinoin and adapalene should not be used for the treatment of acne in pregnancy because of their safety concerns. Although recent studies on topical tretinoin and adapalene have not been associated with a significantly increased risk of birth defects when used after the first trimester of pregnancy.

Oral antibiotics like azithromycin and cephalosporins used for the treatment of acne are pregnancy category B drugs and can be used for the treatment of acne in pregnancy in severe and non responding cases. Oral tetracyclines like doxycycline and lymecycline are pregnancy category D drugs and are associated with congenital abnormalities including deposition of these antibiotics in the dentition and skeletal system leading to growth defects and dental abnormalities of the fetus. Tetracyclines have been associated with these complications especially when used after the first trimester of pregnancy. They should hence be avoided in pregnancy. In case of women of reproductive age group conceives while on treatment with oral tetracyclines these medications should be discontinued as pregnancy is diagnosed (before first trimester) and pregnancy be allowed to continue.

Oral zinc can be given as an adjunct in treatment of acne vulgaris in doses of less than 50 mg per day as low doses of zinc during pregnancy have not been associated with any fetal growth abnormalities.

Other oral medications which are conventionally used in treatment of routine cases of acne vulgaris like oral isotretinoin, spironolactone and OCPs are not recommended to be used in pregnancy. Oral isotretinoin which is a pregnancy category X drug is associated with significant congenital abnormalities and adverse events in the fetus. It has to be strictly avoided in patients who are trying to plan pregnancy or have the potential to become pregnant during the course of treatment.

Physical therapies for the treatment of acne like chemical peels, intra lesional injections and the use of lasers should be deferred during the course of pregnancy.

Rosacea in pregnancy

Rosacea is another common inflammatory disorder affecting the pilosebaceous unit and cutaneous vasculature. It can have a varied presentation characterized by a predominant centrofacial distribution and features ranging from presence of erythema and telangiectasias, papulopustular lesions surrounded by erythema, phymatous changes and ocular involvement.

Etio pathogenesis

It involves the multifactorial interplay of various factors like androgen modulation, role of Toll like receptor-2 (TLR-2) and increased vascular hypersensitivity. The role of an altered innate immune response, neurovascular imbalance and photo exacerbation have also been suggested. Known exacerbating factors include ultraviolet radiation, hot and spicy food, stress, hot weather and organisms like demodex mite. These changes are believed to trigger an inflammatory reaction in the pilosebaceous unit and the dermal vasculature leading to the clinical manifestations seen in rosacea.

Toll-like receptor-2 has been seen to promote the secretion of TNF alpha and interleukin 1 which lead to activation of Th1 and Th17 pathway. The cytokines which are released as a result of activation of these pathways lead to induction of secondary molecules like vascular endothelial growth factor (VEGF) which is believed to play a role in angiogenesis. Ultraviolet radiation is believed to trigger the keratinocytes to produce chemokine ligands like CXCL1 and CXCL8 which facilitate neutrophil chemotaxis.

Clinical features

Rosacea presents with a predominant centrofacial distribution involving the contours of the face because of the predominance of sebaceous glands in these regions. It is broadly classified to be of four subtypes:

- **Erythemato-telangeactatic type:** It is characterized by episodic flushing and telangiectasias in a centrofacial distribution involving the contours of the face with often with sparing of the nasolabial folds.

- **Papulopustular rosacea**: It presents with papules and pustules on the background of erythema however unlike in acne comedonal lesions are not usually seen.

- **Phymatous rosacea:** It presents in the form of diffuse skin thickness and nodularity along with enlargement of the nose known as rhinophyma. Similar changes may also be seen on the forehead, cheeks, chin and the ears.

- **Ocular rosacea:** It can present in the form of eyelid involvement, conjunctivitis, keratitis iridocyclitis and scleritis. It can sometimes prove to be serious and can affect the vision of the patient if not treated correctly.

Rosacea can present in a severe form during pregnancy and is known as **rosacea fulminans (RF)** or pyoderma faciale. It is characterized by development of multiple pustules, abscess and sinuses along with severe facial swelling. RF can be associated with adverse outcomes like IUGR, abortion and preterm delivery. Corneal perforation has also been reported in a case of RF associated with ocular involvement.

Management

General measures like avoidance of triggers including sunlight, hot and spicy food, alcohol, high environmental temperature, smoking and stress should be emphasized.

Papulopustular lesions of rosacea in pregnancy can be treated with azelaic acid, clindamycin or metronidazole which are considered safer for use during pregnancy.

Erythemato-telangeactatic type responds best to the use of vascular lasers however they are better to be avoided until the time of delivery. Mild ocular involvement in rosacea can be treated with erythromycin eye ointment and sulfa eye drops.

Rosacea fulminans in pregnancy should be treated with topical and oral corticosteroids to control the acute flare of the disease. Other medications which have been used in the treatment of RF include oral azithromycin, erythromycin and topical metronidazole.

References

1. Griffith, C. E.M., & Baker, J. (Eds.). (2016). Rook's Textbook of Dermatology (9th ed., Vol. 3). Willey Blackwell.

2. Ingber, A. (2008). Obstetric Dermatology: A Practical Guide. Springer.

3. Tyler, K. H. (Ed.). (2020). Cutaneous Disorders of Pregnancy. Springer International Publishing.

4. Yang CS, Teeple M, Muglia J, Robinson-Bostom L. Inflammatory and glandular skin disease in pregnancy. Clin Dermatol. 2016;34(3):335–43. https://doi.org/10.1016/j.clindermatol.2016.02.005.

5. Ratzer MA. The influence of marriage, pregnancy and childbirth on acne vulgaris. Br J Dermatol. 1964;76:165-168.

6. Shaw JC, White LE. Persistent acne in adult women. Arch Dermatol. 2001;137:1252-1253..

7. Van Pelt HP, Juhlin L. Acne conglobata after pregnancy. Acta Derm Venereol. 1999;79:169.

8. Akhavan A, Bershad S. Topical acne drugs: Review of clinical properties, systemic exposure, and safety. Am J Clin Dermatol. 2003;4:473-492.

9. Mylonas I. Antibiotic chemotherapy during pregnancy and lactation period: Aspects for consideration. Arch Gynecol Obstet. 2011;283:7-18.

10. Culp B, Scheinfeld N. Rosacea: A review. P T. 2009;34:38-45.

11. Cribier B. Pathophysiology of rosacea: Redness, telangiectasia and rosacea. Ann Dermatol Venereol. 2011;138:184-191.

12. Jarrett R, Gonsalves R, Anstey AV. Differing obstetric outcomes of rosacea fulminans in pregnancy: Report of three cases with review of pathogenesis and management. Clin Exp Dermatol. 2010;35:888-891.

13. Goldgar C, Keahey DJ, Houchins J. Treatment options for acne rosacea. Am Fam Physician. 2009;80:461-468.

14. Jansen T, Plewig G, KligmanAM. Diagnosis and treatment of rosacea fulminans. Dermatology. 1994;188:251-254.

Chapter 13

Diseases Of The Apocrine And Eccrine Glands In Pregnancy

Apocrine Gland Diseases in Pregnancy

The activity of apocrine glands during pregnancy is shown to be decreased. These disorders which involve the apocrine glands like the Fox Fordyce disease (FFD) and Hidradenitis suppurativa (HS) show temporary remission during pregnancy. Both the diseases are seen to rebound after delivery due to the recovery in activity of apocrine glands in the postpartum period.

Hidradenitis suppurativa (HS)

Hidradenitis suppurativa is a chronic inflammatory dermatoses that predominantly affects the apocrine gland bearing areas like the axilla, inguinal region, perineum, perianal region and the inframammary area. It is characterized by development of recurrent papulonodular lesions, pustules, cystic abscesses and draining sinuses along with induration and scarring. Most cases develop after puberty and it is more common in females as compared to males. The data regarding the effect of pregnancy on hidradenitis suppurativa has been conflicting with some studies showing improvement and stabilization of disease in HS while others showing exacerbation. Although, it is conventionally believed that apocrine gland activity decreases during pregnancy and consequently HS should also improve during pregnancy. However, the role of weight gain and sweating seen in pregnancy may be responsible for worsening of HS due to increased skin maceration. Also, increase in the production of TNF alpha secretion by adipocytes can contribute to worsening of HS in pregnancy. On the other hand, progesterone increase during pregnancy is believed to decrease HS severity because of its anti-inflammatory effects.

Management of HS includes general measures like wearing of loose fitting cotton clothes to avoid triggering factors like sweating, shaving of hair, smoking etc. Conservative treatment in the form of topical therapy with safe agents like clindamycin is usually preferred. Intra lesional corticosteroid injections can be given in isolated nodulocystic lesions. Safe oral antibiotics like oral macrolides and clindamycin can be used in severe cases during pregnancy. Use of biologicals and surgical modalities during pregnancy is usually reserved for refractory cases only.

Fox Fordyce disease (FFD)

Fox fordyce disease is another apocrine gland disorder caused by the blockage of infundibular opening of the follicle due to accumulation of keratin leading to obstruction of the apocrine gland secretion. Clinically it presents in the form of multiple small monomorphic papules in the axilla, groins and mammary region predominantly in females of reproductive age group. FFD is believed to improve during the course of pregnancy due to decrease in apocrine gland activity.

Management of FFD during pregnancy includes the use of topical antibiotics, mild topical steroids and UVB light therapy. Oral and surgical modalities using OCPs and spironolactone are usually not required and avoided during pregnancy.

Eccrine Glands Diseases in Pregnancy

Hyperhidrosis

Hyperhidrosis is defined as excessive sweating beyond what is normally required for thermoregulation. Pregnancy is associated with increased activity of eccrine glands especially during the third trimester. Hyperhidrosis in pregnancy can be managed with topical aluminum hexachloride solution which has to be applied once everyday before going to bed. Other modalities of treatment of hyperhidrosis like iontophoresis, botulinum toxin injections, oral glycopyrrolate and oxybutynin are avoided during pregnancy and lactation.

Miliaria

Increased sweating seen due to overactivity of eccrine glands during pregnancy can lead to a condition called as miliaria which is caused by occlusion of ducts of eccrine glands (sweat glands). Miliaria can present in different forms depending upon the level of occlusion of the eccrine duct. These include miliaria crystallina, miliaria rubra and miliaria profunda. Other factors which can contribute to the development of miliaria include hot and humid climate, obesity and hyperthyroidism.

Treatment of miliaria in pregnancy includes avoidance of hot and humid climate, wearing light coloured cotton clothes, clothing should be loose and non occlusive, and taking frequent showers. Non occlusive moisturizers with anti pruritic compounds like menthol and calamine can be applied for symptomatic relief. First generation oral antihistamines can be used for alleviation of pruritus.

References

1. Ingber, A. (2008). Obstetric Dermatology: A Practical Guide. Springer.

2. Tyler, K. H. (Ed.). (2020). Cutaneous Disorders of Pregnancy. Springer International Publishing.

3. Miller JL, Hurley HJ. Diseases of the eccrine and apocrine sweat glands. In: Bolognia JL, Jorizzo JL, Rapini RP, eds. Dermatology. 2nd ed. Philadelphia, PA: Mosby Elsevier; 2008. p. 531-548.

4. Oumeish OY, Al-Fouzan AW (2006) Miscellaneous diseases affected by pregnancy. Clin Dermatol 24:113–117

5. Alikhan A, Lynch PJ, Eisen DB. Hidradenitis suppurativa: A comprehensive review. J AmAcad Dermatol. 2009;60:539-561.

6. Fernandez JM, Hendricks AJ, Thompson AM, et al. Menses, pregnancy, delivery, and menopause in hidradenitis suppurativa: A patient survey. Int J Womens Dermatol. 2020;6(5):368-371. Published 2020 Jul 10.

   doi:10.1016/j.ijwd.2020.07.002

7. Plagens-Rotman K, Przybylska R, Gerke K, et al. Acute form of acne inversa in an 18-week pregnant patient: a case study. Postepy Dermatol Alergol. 2019;36(2):242-246.

   doi:10.5114/ada.2018.79472

8. Montero-Vilchez T, Salvador-Rodriguez L, Rodriguez-Tejero A, Sanchez-Diaz M, Arias-Santiago S, Molina-Leyva A. Reproductive Potential and Outcomes in Patients with Hidradenitis Suppurativa: Clinical Profile and Therapeutic Implications. Life. 2021; 11(4):277.

https://doi.org/10.3390/life11040277

9. Kronthal HL, Pomeranz JR, Stiomer G. Fox-Fordyce disease: Treatment with an oral contraceptive. Arch Dermatol. 1965;91:243-245.

10. Pradhan S, Madke B, Sirka CS. Review of oral anticholinergics in the treatment of palmoplantar hyperhidrosis. Indian J Drugs Dermatol 2019;5:75-82

Chapter 14

Metabolic Diseases In Pregnancy

Pregnancy is characterized by marked changes in the hormonal, immunological and metabolic system of the female body. Metabolic disorders such as Porphyria cutanea tarda and acrodermatitis enteropathica show significant exacerbation during the course of pregnancy. While exaggeration seen in porphyria cutanea tarda can occur both during pregnancy and the postpartum period, the increase in severity of acrodermatitis enteropathica is usually limited to the period of pregnancy only.

Porphyria cutanea tarda (PCT)

PCT is the most common of all the types of porphyrias. It can be familial or hereditary and sporadic or acquired. Seventy five percent of patients of PCT suffer from type 1 PCT which is sporadic in nature usually presenting in the later years of life. It is a relatively milder version of porphyria and the enzyme deficiency is present in the liver only; often uncovered due to extrinsic insults. Iron overload in the liver is often seen due to defective erythropoiesis. Haemochromatosis is the most common cause of iron overload associated with sporadic PCT. The milder presentation of sporadic PCT is believed to be due to heterozygosity of haemochromatosis alleles.

Type 2 PCT is familial type and the enzyme deficiency is present in all the tissues. The mode of inheritance of familial PCT is autosomal dominant with low penetrance. Thus family history may not be present in all cases of type 2 PCT. Clinical features usually initiate at an early age of around 20 years as compared to around 40 to 50 years of age in type 1 PCT.

Etiopathogenesis

PCT is caused due to the deficiency of an enzyme namely **uroporphyrinogen decarboxylase (UROD)** which is an important enzyme in the heme synthesis pathway. Deficiency of UROD enzyme leads to abnormal accumulation of porphyrin compounds, mainly uroporphyrins. Porphyrins are endogenously produced photosensitizers and are responsible for the photodamage seen in porphyrias.

Clinical presentation

Both sporadic and familial types of PCT present with similar clinical features in the form of photosensitivity, blisters, pigmentary changes, scarring and hypertrichosis more so in a photo distributed pattern especially involving dorsum of the hands and scalp. Blisters are often tense and rupture on manipulation to form erosions and crust which later heal with pigmentary changes, scarring and millia formation. There is also an increased fragility of the skin as it is prone to get damaged on trivial trauma. Scarring alopecia and pseudo sclerodermatous changes in the skin may develop in the later stages of the disease. Systemic involvement may lead to development of liver enlargement, cirrhosis and diabetes mellitus. Both types of PCT are exacerbated on exposure to external triggers like estrogen, hepatitis C infection, alcohol intake, iron intake and use of hepatotoxic drugs.

Because of pregnancy being a hyper oestrogenic state PCT usually aggravates during the course of pregnancy and postpartum period. Exacerbation seen with intake of oral contraceptive pills is also attributed to the role of hormones, especially estrogen. Many studies have reported disease exacerbations during the period of pregnancy along with increased excretion of plasma and urine porphyrins during this period. The disease exacerbation is usually maximum during the first trimester of pregnancy due to the rise of estrogen levels during this period. During the second and third trimester the disease severity lessens due to the effect of hemodilution, increased requirement of blood and iron by the fetus along with decrease in levels of estrogen and progesterone as the pregnancy progresses. It is seen that PCT normally decreases in intensity as the pregnancy passes from the first trimester to the second and third trimester. Use of drugs like barbiturates, antifungals and antituberculars is associated with worsening of PCT.

PCT itself mein have deleterious effects on the course of pregnancy. Liver involvement in PCT may cause elevation of liver enzymes. Patients with PCT have a high risk of hepatitis B and C infection hence any pregnant female coming with PCT should be tested for viral antibodies and antigens and special care should be taken by the staff while handling the mother and the baby in such cases. Patients of PCT can also present with diabetes or impaired glucose tolerance and should be screened for fasting blood sugar levels. Some patients of PCT may test positive for antinuclear antibodies and anticardiolipin antibodies. PCT patients during pregnancy are prone to develop preeclampsia and its complications. Hence, it is advisable to start low dose aspirin in cases of PCT with pregnancy testing positive for anticardiolipin antibodies to avoid fetal loss and thrombotic complications. Some reports also suggest an increased incidence of HIV infection in patients of PCT.

The data accessing effects of PCT on fetal outcomes per se is scanty. However it is a good practice to assess the neonate and screen for the presence of PCT in neonate. The evidence to suggest any harmful effects of breastfeeding in infants of mothers suffering from PCT is inadequate.

Histopathology

The blisters in PCT show subepidermal level of split and the dermal papillae appear to invaginate within the blister cavity which is known as *festoning*. Eosinophilic bodies may be demonstrated extending from the roof of blisters which are known as *caterpillar bodies*. Direct immunofluorescence studies show deposition of immune reactants IgG and C3 at the level of the basement membrane and around the dermal blood vessels.

Diagnosis

The diagnosis of porphyria cutanea tarda is made on clinical grounds and histopathological findings. Porphyrin analysis should be done when available to differentiate PCT from other types of porphyrias. Urine analysis for porphyrins in PCT shows increased levels of uroporphyrins and hepatoporphyrins. Plasma and stool analysis also shows increased porphyrin levels. A simple bedside test to demonstrate porphyrins in urine is by wood's lamp examination of the urine which gives pink red fluorescence.

Treatment

General measures in the form of strict photoprotection and use of a good sunscreen preferably physical sunscreen are advised in all patients. Oral drug therapy in PCT consists of low dose hydroxychloroquine or chloroquine given in twice weekly doses. Phlebotomy is usually done weekly or biweekly to drain around 500 ml of venous blood in each sitting in order to prevent iron overload. Clinical improvement usually takes 2 to 3 months. The goal of venesection is to keep plasma ferritin levels less than 25 microgram per liter and hemoglobin at the level of 10-11 grams per deciliter. Management in relation to pregnancy includes avoidance of known triggers like alcohol, sun exposure, drugs and oral iron. PCT usually improves during the later half of pregnancy after the first trimester is over. Hydroxychloroquine and phlebotomy are both considered to be relatively safe in pregnancy and can be taken as treatment modalities in cases where the disease is severe or not improving even after completion of the first trimester of pregnancy. There is no indication of doing a cesarean section in cases of PCT per se. However if a cesarean section is required for any other indication it can be undertaken after a complete pre-anesthetic check up. Administration of general or regional anesthesia in such patients has not been associated with adverse events.

Acrodermatitis Enteropathica (AE)

Acrodermatitis enteropathica is an autosomal recessive disorder characterized by the presence of dermatitis involving the acral and periorificial areas. The most common age group affected by acrodermatitis enteropathica is infants and children.

Etiopathogenesis

Acrodermatitis enteropathica is an autosomal recessive disorder caused due to the mutation in zinc transporter protein HZip 4. The condition arises due to a state of zinc deficiency caused by impaired gastrointestinal absorption of zinc.

Clinical presentation

The patients suffering from AE present with acral and periorificial involvement characterized by blisters, oozy erosions and crust formation. Milder variants of AE may present with involvement of acral sites only. This is often associated with extracutaneous symptoms in the form of chronic diarrhea and hair loss which is more common in childhood AE. Severe cases of AE suffer from recurrent infections, failure to thrive, loss of appetite, hypogonadism and can even cause death.

Flare up of AE or reappearance of AE may occur during the pregnancy because of decrease in the blood zinc levels as a result of increased demand of zinc during pregnancy. Besides increased demand of zinc during pregnancy, estrogen hormone has also been attributed to play a role in the acrodermatitis enteropathica in pregnancy. In AE the patient usually presents with a history of mild non specific skin lesions predominantly acral and periorificial in distribution occurring for the first time during childhood which usually subside after puberty.

In some cases it is seen to reappear during pregnancy. AE during pregnancy usually appears in the first or early second trimester and keeps on worsening until delivery, followed by remission in the postpartum period. Some studies have reported the occurrence of congenital abnormalities in newborns of mothers suffering from acrodermatitis enteropathica.

Differential diagnosis

Acrodermatitis enteropathica can be confused with other dermatoses presenting with oozy erosions and blisters during pregnancy such as pemphigoid gestationis, generalized pustular psoriasis of pregnancy, infected eczemas and irritant contact dermatitis. In doubtful cases plasma zinc levels can be measured to confirm the diagnosis of AE.

Diagnosis

Diagnosis is primarily made on the basis of clinical presentation and age group distribution. It can be confirmed by assessing the levels of zinc in the plasma or serum.

Treatment

Oral zinc in the form of zinc sulfate, zinc acetate or zinc gluconate is commonly available in the market and any preparation providing 30 to 50 mg of elemental zinc daily can reverse the manifestations of AE within days. Zinc is safe to be administered in doses of less than 50 milligram of elemental zinc daily and is not known to cause any teratogenic side effects. Cases of AE trying to conceive, can be started prophylactically on zinc supplementation so as to avoid exacerbation of the disease during pregnancy and prevent chances of developing congenital abnormalities in the fetus.

References

1. Ingber, A. (2008). Obstetric Dermatology: A Practical Guide. Springer.

2. Perez-Maldonado A, Kurban AK (2006) Metabolic diseases and pregnancy. Clin Dermatol 24:88–90

3. Winton GB. Skin diseases aggravated by pregnancy. J Am Acad Dermatol 1989;20:1 - 13.

4. Aziz Ibrahim A, Esen UI (2004) Porphyria cutanea tarda in pregnancy: a case report. J Obstet Gynaecol 24:574–575

5. Mital TK, Fuke RP. Pregnancy in porphyria and its complications: a case report. Int J Reprod Contracept Obstet Gynecol 2020;9:4722-5.

6. Tollånes MC, Aarsand AK, Sandberg S. Excess risk of adverse pregnancy outcomes in women with porphyria: a population-based cohort study. J Inherit Metab Dis. 2011;34(1):217-223. doi:10.1007/s10545-010-9231-2

7. Saritha M, Gupta D, Chandrashekar L, Thappa DM, Rajesh NG. Acquired zinc deficiency in an adult female. Indian J Dermatol. 2012;57(6):492-494. doi:10.4103/0019-5154.103073

8. Verburg DJ, Burd LI, Hoxtell EO, Merrill LK. Acrodermatitis enteropathica and pregnancy. Obstet Gynecol. 1974 Aug;44(2):233-7. PMID: 4607826.

Chapter 15

Structural Connective Tissue Diseases In Pregnancy

Introduction

Connective tissue of human skin is made up of fibers including collagen and elastin enmeshed within an amorphous ground substance. Any structural defect in these components can present as a connective tissue disorder which can be congenital or acquired. Collagen which forms the majority component of connective tissue can be affected in connective tissue disorders like Ehler Danlos Syndrome. Elastic fibers can be affected in disorders like anetoderma, cutis laxa and pseudoxanthoma elasticum. Because of the changes in cutaneous and subcutaneous tissues which occur during pregnancy the integrity of connective tissue is challenged by the course of pregnancy. Hence, structural connective tissue disorders become relevant in the relation with pregnancy. In this chapter we shall discuss some important structural connective tissue disorders which hold relevance in the context of pregnancy.

Pseudoxanthoma elasticum (PXE)

Etiopathogenesis

It is a progressive genetic disorder, usually autosomal recessive disorder (90%) and autosomal dominant in others characterized by abnormal calcification of elastic fibers affecting the connective tissue structure of skin, retina and the vascular tissue of the gastrointestinal, cardiovascular and genitourinary system. The arteries of the gastrointestinal, cardiovascular and urogenital system can undergo calcification of the internal elastic lamina leading to impairment of their elasticity, narrowing of the vascular lumen, damage to the vessels and consequent hemorrhages presenting as gastrointestinal bleeding and haematuria. The phenomenon of vascular calcification is also seen in the coronary vessels which can present with adverse cardiovascular outcomes like myocardial infarction and angina. Mutation of the ABCC6 gene which is located on chromosome 16 is believed to be responsible for the causation of PXE.

Clinical presentation

PXE is a genetic disease characterized by vascular calcification affecting various organs like the skin, eyes, gastrointestinal system, cardiovascular system and genito-urinary system. The cutaneous lesions are usually first seen during or after puberty and are characterized by the development of pale to yellowish papules and plaques studded over a lax and redundant skin giving a typical "plucked chicken skin appearance" in the areas of body folds like the neck, axillary region and inguinal region.

Ocular manifestations present predominantly in the form of *angioid streaks* which are seen due to calcification of bruch's membrane in the retina. They are usually asymptomatic and are often encountered during ocular follow up of PXE patients. During the later stages retinal involvement may present as retinal hemorrhage or detachment. Gastrointestinal and genitourinary bleeding are less commonly seen.

PXE and pregnancy

The older literature has suggested the possibility of maternal and fetal complications primarily in the form of maternal gastrointestinal bleeding and fetal issues. Many conventional authors have advocated against conception in patients of PXE and have indicated adverse pregnancy outcomes in such patients.

The possibility of transmission of disease to the fetus due to the PXE being a hereditary disease has been a major deterrent for a parent suffering from PXE to undergo pregnancy. This was further compounded by the fare of adverse pregnancy outcomes including maternal hemorrhages and fetal complications as well as chances of pregnancy exacerbating the disease severity of PXE in the mother. The main complications reported in these studies included higher chances of gastrointestinal hemorrhage, worsening of cutaneous lesions, hypertension and vascular thrombosis. Some previous studies have also reported adverse fetal complications like intrauterine growth retardation due to the calcification of placental tissue.

Studies published recently have suggested that patients suffering from PXE do not necessarily carry significant risk of pregnancy as suggested by older literature. These studies have suggested that complications of PXE in mothers like gastric bleeding and retinal complications were actually less common than what were believed to be.

As far as the effect of PXE in pregnancy on the fetus was concerned, Newer studies revealed that the calcification of placental tissue did not have a significant effect on the impairment of fetomaternal transport of nutrients. Majority of pregnancies with PXE were uncomplicated and no fetal complications were seen. However the most common complication reported in the studies was an increase in cutaneous complications which were seen in 12% of the cases followed by hypertension which was seen in 10%. However these changes were usually benign and did not affect the mother or child critically.

Overall it seems that the patients suffering from PXE do not carry a higher risk of complications in comparison to non pregnant patients. However at the same time it is prudent that the patients of PXE in pregnancy should be monitored for gastrointestinal, retinal and skin complications as for non pregnant PXE patients. Most of the patients of PXE who underwent pregnancy give birth to healthy babies without significant complications.

Anetoderma

The word anetoderma is derived from two Greek words *anetos* which means loose and *derma* which means skin. It is a condition which is primarily caused due to the defect of elastic fibers in the connective tissue. It can be primary in which there is no inflammatory trigger causing anetoderma and secondary where anetoderma is caused by an inflammatory condition like lupus or acne or syphilis.

Primary anetoderma is further divided into two types:

Jadassohn-Pellizari type in which the preceding lesions are urticarial whereas in Schweninger-Buzzi type the lesions occur on normal skin. Anetoderma can also occur secondary to the use of drugs or maybe associated with prematurity.

Clinical features

Clinically anetoderma presents as multiple skin coloured to whiteish, well defined, round to oval lesions characterized by cutaneous atrophy and herniation of the subcutaneous fat. The most common sites involved include the trunk and limbs.

Anetoderma and pregnancy

Whether primary anetoderma has an effect on pregnancy is not clear. However in cases of secondary anetoderma causes like lupus and syphilis should be ruled out and patients should be screened for anticardiolipin antibodies and vdrl in suspected cases.

Treatment for anetoderma is not established hence watchful expectancy is all that is needed in cases of anetoderma in pregnancy.

Ehler Danlos Syndrome (EDS)

It is a hereditary disorder characterized by defects in the collagen fibers of connective tissue predominantly affecting the skin and joints. The clinical presentation and pattern of genetic defect can be varied. It is divided into 6 types out of which type 1, 2 and 3 are the most common.

Clinical presentation

EDS is characterized clinically by the presence of joint hypermobility, hyper extensibility and easy fragility of the skin. Depending upon the predominant presentation EDS has been classified into 6 different types. Type four EDS also known as the vascular type has the worst prognosis characterized by vascular complications in the form of vascular rupture and hemorrhage involving the large arteries.

Ehler Danlos Syndrome and pregnancy

There have been reports of adverse maternal and fetal complications in patients of EDS during pregnancy. Exacerbation of the disease has also been reported in the mothers during pregnancy. Worsening of the joint symptoms in these patients is the most common presentation. Fetal complications like premature delivery and abortions have been reported due to the cervical incompetence seen during early phases of pregnancy. Other complications which have been reported in cases of EDS in pregnancy include premature rupture of membranes, scar dehiscence after cesarean section, hernia, hemorrhages and hematomas.

The risk to the mother includes the chances of arterial rupture and hemorrhage involving the aorta and uterine artery especially during the time of delivery. Other possible complications which can arise in the mother suffering from EDS include chances of perineal tears, thus instrumental delivery should be avoided. Possibility of atonic postpartum hemorrhage, delayed wound healing and atrophic scars also exist.

Fetal complications are usually less common than the maternal complications and include intrauterine growth retardation and floppy infant syndrome.

Recent studies suggest that patients with hypermobility EDS who got pregnant generally had a fair prognosis however in those with vascular type of EDS where arterial complications tend to happen have a bad maternal prognosis.

Patients of Ehler Danlos Syndrome during pregnancy should be monitored for maternal and fetal complications. Cesarean section delivery is not mandatory in all cases. Normal vaginal route of delivery should be tried in cases with no obstetric contraindications. Cesarean should be done only in high risk cases and in those with severe joint complications like hip dislocation. Possibility of quick labor and atonic postpartum hemorrhage should be kept in mind. Prompt episiotomy should be done in order to avoid perineal trauma during labor.

References

1. Ingber, A. (2008). Obstetric Dermatology: A Practical Guide. Springer.

2. Tyler, K. H. (Ed.). (2020). Cutaneous Disorders of Pregnancy. Springer International Publishing.

3. Lee R, Lebwohl M. Comprehensive Literature Review of Obstetric Outcomes and Fetal Risk during Pregnancy with Pseudoxanthoma Elasticum. J Clin Med. 2021 Jun 7;10(11):2532. doi: 10.3390/jcm10112532. PMID: 34200486; PMCID: PMC8201327.

4. Bercovitch L, Leroux T, Terry S, Weinstock MA. Pregnancy and obstetrical outcomes in pseudoxanthoma elasticum. Br J Dermatol. 2004 Nov;151(5):1011-8. doi: 10.1111/j.1365-2133.2004.06183.x. PMID: 15541079.

5. Berde, Charles; Willis, Donald C.; Sandberg, Eugene C.. Pregnancy in Women with Pseudoxanthoma Elasticum. Obstetrical & Gynecological Survey 38(6):p 339-344, June 1983.

6. Ramos-E-Silva M, Líbia Cardozo Pereira A, Bastos Oliveira G, Coelho da Silva Carneiro S. Connective tissue diseases: pseudoxanthoma elasticum, anetoderma, and Ehlers-Danlos syndrome in pregnancy. Clin Dermatol. 2006 Mar-Apr;24(2):91-6. doi: 10.1016/j.clindermatol.2005.10.005. PMID: 16487880.

7. Karthikeyan A, Venkat-Raman N. Hypermobile Ehlers-Danlos syndrome and pregnancy. *Obstet Med.* 2018;11(3):104-109. doi:10.1177/1753495X18754577

8. Kang J, Hanif M, Mirza E, Jaleel S. Ehlers-Danlos Syndrome in Pregnancy: A Review. Eur J Obstet Gynecol Reprod Biol. 2020 Dec;255:118-123. doi: 10.1016/j.ejogrb.2020.10.033. Epub 2020 Oct 17. PMID: 33113401.

Chapter 16

Uncommon Conditions Associated with Pregnancy

Autoimmune Progesterone Dermatitis In Pregnancy

Autoimmune progesterone dermatitis (APD) of pregnancy is a rare condition described in only a few cases characterized by the development of a symptomatic acral eruption caused due to hypersensitivity to progesterone.

Etiopathogenesis

The appearance of skin lesions during pregnancy and on use of oral contraceptive pills containing progesterone, reappearance of localized lesions on giving intradermal progesterone injection and improvement in the lesions on applying conjugated estrogen, support the role of progesterone in causation of autoimmune progesterone dermatitis. Similar lesions have also been reported in pre and post menopausal women. Cultures taken from the skin of patients suffering from autoimmune progesterone dermatitis have revealed growth of *Proteus, Klebsiella* and *Enterobacter;* while samples taken from the pustular lesions grew *E. coli* and *Staphylococcus aureus* on culture.

Clinical presentation

The rash of autoimmune progesterone dermatitis in pregnancy starts within weeks of conception in the form of follicular papules and pustules involving the acral areas. The papules are usually subcentimeter in size, often tender and grouped in distribution. Vesiculation which is a hallmark of APD in non pregnant cases is not usually seen with autoimmune progesterone dermatitis of pregnancy. However pustules present on an inflammatory base and containing turbid fluid are often seen during the later course of disease in pregnancy. The lesions often heal with post inflammatory hyperpigmentation. In APD of pregnancy the lesions are mostly distributed on the acral sites especially the fingers, arms, legs and buttocks. This is followed by the appearance of papulosquamous lesions with psoriasiform scales. The skin lesions are also associated with joint involvement in the form of polyarticular arthritis. Polyarthritis seen in APD of pregnancy commonly involves the smaller joints of hands, wrist joint, knees and ankle joint. Autoimmune progesterone dermatitis of pregnancy can reoccur with subsequent pregnancies.

In the two cases reported, it was seen to be associated with spontaneous abortion in both cases; after which the lesions settled down gradually.

In non pregnant cases of APD, the entity is much more well understood. It is characterized by the appearance of rash consisting of urticarial wheals and bullous lesions developing on the trunk and acral extremities. The rash tends to reappear a week before menstruation during each menstrual cycle. It has also been seen in association with intake of progesterone containing hormonal pills. The disease has shown improvement with estrogen therapy and surgical oophorectomy.

Intradermal skin tests with progesterone are often positive. A positive intradermal test is interpreted as development of a pustular lesions and abscess at the site of progesterone injection 48 hours after the test. Immunofluorescence studies were found to be negative.

Histopathology

Skin biopsy of the lesions showed epidermal changes in the form of acanthosis, focal spongiosis and exocytosis of lymphocytes and histiocytes. A moderately dense infiltrate of eosinophils was seen interspersed in the dermis and in the perivascular region. Subcutaneous tissue showed the presence of lobular panniculitis with the presence of eosinophils, lymphocytes and histiocytes along with eosinophilic abscess formation.

Differential diagnosis

Other diseases which can present with a papulopustular eruption during pregnancy should be excluded. These conditions include acneiform drug eruptions, acne fulminans and iododermas. The presence of typical acral distribution and positive intradermal progesterone test are characteristic of autoimmune progesterone dermatitis. Due to the rare occurrence of autoimmune progesterone dermatitis in pregnancy, it should always be a diagnosis of exclusion.

Treatment

There is no proven treatment of autoimmune progesterone dermatitis in pregnancy and the only option available is watchful expectancy and monitoring the fetus for any adverse outcomes. In non pregnant autoimmune progesterone dermatitis associated with premenstrual flares, the aim of treatment is to suppress progesterone surge seen during ovulation. For this, ovulation inhibition is done using 1.25 mg conjugated equine estrogen given daily for 21 days in a month.

Linear IgM dermatoses (LID) of pregnancy

Clinical presentation

It presents in the form of itchy red follicular papules and pustules over the abdomen and the extremities. The rash typically does not respond to oral antihistamines and topical calamine lotion. Only a few case reports exist till date which describe linear IgM dermatoses of pregnancy to appear during the third trimester of pregnancy around the time of delivery and after delivery it tends to resolve within 1 to 2 months.

Investigations

Skin biopsy done from the lesion shows features resembling folliculitis. Direct immunofluorescence study reveals deposition of IgM at the level of basement membrane in a linear fashion. Indirect immunofluorescence study is negative. Circulating IgM antibodies against basement membrane zone in indirect immunofluorescence studies have been shown in healthy pregnant females and in other conditions like polymorphic eruption of pregnancy.

Diagnosis

IgM deposition at the level of dermo-epidermal junction has also been seen in men and non pregnant females; as well as in other conditions like vasculitis, urticaria, folliculitis, pigmented purpuric disease etc. Because of these findings, it is difficult to determine if linear IgM disease of pregnancy is a separate entity in itself or a manifestation of some pregnancy associated dermatoses like PEP. Overall, the rash of LID is not known to affect the pregnancy outcome.

References

1. Bierman SM. Autoimmune Progesterone Dermatitis of Pregnancy. Arch Dermatol. 1973;107(6):896–901. doi:10.1001/archderm.1973.01620210060016

2. Kanninen TT, Moretti ML, Lakhi NA. Autoimmune progesterone dermatitis following vaginal progesterone exposure in pregnancy. Obstet Med. 2019;12(2):100-102. doi:10.1177/1753495X18771255

3. Yavuz AF, Akcay GFY, Kara H, Tas EE, Keskin HL. Autoimmune Progesterone Dermatitis during Pregnancy Results in a Full-Term Delivery. J Clin Med Case Reports. 2016;3(1): 3.

4. Joseph Alcalay, Arieh Ingber, Bilha Hazaz, Michael David, Miriam Sandbank, Linear IgM dermatoses of pregnancy, Journal of the American Academy of Dermatology, Volume 18, Issue 2, Part 2, 1988, Pages 412-415,

5. Velthuis PJ, de Jong MC, Kruis MH (1988) Is there a linear IgM dermatoses? Significance of linear IgM junctional staining in cutaneous immunopathology. Acta Derm Venereol 68:8–14

Chapter 17

Neoplastic Conditions In Pregnancy

Non-Melanoma Skin Cancers (NMSCs)

Non-melanoma skin cancers like basal cell carcinoma and squamous cell carcinoma are the most common types of skin cancers. There is some evidence of increased mucosal site squamous cell carcinomas occurring during pregnancy involving various mucosal sites like the oral mucosa, tongue, vulva and the cervix. There are reports of basal cell carcinomas occurring during pregnancy which may show an unusual and aggressive behavior. However there is no concrete data to suggest the definite association of non melanoma skin cancers with pregnancy.

Severe neoplastic conditions like Merkel cell carcinoma and dermatofibrosarcoma protuberans (DFSP), if occurring during pregnancy should be treated aggressively and early without waiting for completion of pregnancy due to chances of rapid metastasis.

Malignant Melanoma (MM)

Changes in melanocytic lesions in pregnancy

There is an increased tendency of hyperpigmentation in pregnancy due to the stimulation of melanocyte stimulating hormone by estrogen and progesterone. Pigmented lesions like freckles, lentigines and melanocytic nevi may show physiological increase in pigmentation which can be misinterpreted as dysplastic change. However in most of the females this change appears to be physiological and harmless. The changes occurring in melanocytic nevi during pregnancy are often transient and the appearance returns back to its original form after childbirth in majority of the cases. However, sudden change in color or morphology of any nevus during pregnancy should alert the physician and biopsy can be taken to rule out malignant change. In females who have a known history of dysplastic nevus transformation, special care should be taken to evaluate any alteration in color or morphology of the nevi.

Malignant melanoma in pregnancy

Due to the modern lifestyle and females delaying their pregnancy to a later age of 30 to 40 years; the incidence of malignancies associated with pregnancy has increased. Development of malignant melanoma during pregnancy is a bad prognostic sign and is often associated with poor survival rate and early metastasis. The hormonal and immunological alterations which take place during pregnancy make it a state of relative immune suppression. While these changes are aimed at prevention of fetal rejection, the suppression of cell mediated immunity may itself play a role in the development or progression of melanoma. Studies suggest that there may be a delay in diagnosis of malignant melanoma during pregnancy. Some reports suggest that in pregnancy, malignant melanoma tends to follow an aggressive course characterized by higher tendency of bleeding, ulceration, and increase in thickness. However, recent studies have refuted any significant association of malignant melanoma with the course of pregnancy. Thus the available data is conflicting and not adequate to accept or reject the role of hormones and immune changes in pregnancy in the causation of melanomas. Important complication of malignant melanoma in pregnancy is the fetoplacental metastasis seen in advanced cases of metastatic malignant melanoma. Thus during delivery it is important to examine the placenta and the umbilical cord for any evidence of metastasis. In case malignant melanoma metastatises to the fetus, liver involvement is most commonly seen.

Management

The principle of management for malignant melanoma in pregnancy remains the same as in routine cases of malignant melanoma. A suspicious lesion should be biopsied and excision with adequate margin should be done in cases of malignant melanoma. Surgical excision of melanoma in pregnant females is usually a safe procedure and can be done under local anesthesia. In superficial lesions of melanoma measuring less than 1 mm in thickness, a margin of at least 1 cm should be kept whereas in medium thickness lesions measuring 1-4 mm, a surgical margin of at least 2 cm should be kept. In cases of tumor thickness measuring 1-4 mm, sentinel lymph node biopsy can also be undertaken. In advanced cases of malignant melanoma in pregnancy, chemotherapy has also been tried after the first trimester and was found to be relatively safe in terms of fetal outcome. Targeted therapy and immunotherapy are being used more nowadays because of their better safety profile.

Neurofibromatosis

Pregnancy has been associated with the appearance of neurofibromas de-novo or with increase in the size and number of pre-existing neurofibromas. Some of these lesions tend to regress after delivery. Rarely, complications in neurofibromas may arise during pregnancy which may include extensive hemorrhage within the neurofibromas leading to acute blood loss or paralysis occurring due to rapid enlargement of a plexiform neurofibroma. Increase in size of neurofibromas during pregnancy may cause extrinsic compression of vessel walls leading to rupture of large arteries like the renal artery and thoracic arteries. This can manifest in the form of shock and hemothorax although such findings are rare. The incidence of hypertension in cases of neurofibromas in pregnancy is fairly common, however the exact cause responsible for this phenomenon is unknown.

During the course of pregnancy, such cases of neurofibromatosis should be carefully screened and followed up for progression of neurofibromas and its complications.

Other tumorous growths in pregnancy

There is evidence of development of various tumorous growth during pregnancy like **dermatofibromas** which may develop during pregnancy or show increase in the size of pre-existing lesions.

Leiomyomas seem to become larger in size and more painful due to the course of pregnancy. A similar change has been reported in keloids during the period of pregnancy.

A more aggressive tumor known as **dermatofibrosarcoma protuberans** has also been reported to show rapid growth during the period of pregnancy. The rapid growth of dermatofibrosarcoma protuberans was believed to be due to the effect of platelet derived growth factor and progesterone hormone, the levels of which rise during pregnancy.

Similarly, other locally aggressive tumors like **desmoid tumors** can also arise or increase in size during pregnancy and these may require timely intervention in the form of local excision during the pregnancy itself.

Kaposi sarcoma (KS) in pregnancy has been reported to remit, appear de novo and even spread during the course of pregnancy. Some studies have indicated that vascular endothelial growth factor, the level of which is raised in pregnancy, may contribute to the spread of kaposi sarcoma. KS which is asymptomatic and localized to the skin can be managed by watchful expectancy during the pregnancy and treatment can be started after delivery. KS with aggressive course and systemic environment is often associated with HIV infection. These cases may often require aggressive treatment. After delivery, the neonate should be examined to rule out transplacental transmission of HHV8.

Mycosis fungoides is a primary T cell cutaneous non hodgkin lymphoma that is rarely seen in pregnancy. There is no data to suggest its association with pregnancy, except a few case reports showing disease exacerbation during pregnancy which was attributed to a Th2 pathway shift in the immunity.

Angiolymphoid hyperplasia with eosinophilia (ALHE) is a rare tumor associated with blood eosinophilia. An increase in the size of ALHE, appearance of new lesions and even remission has been reported during the course of pregnancy. Lesions of ALHE have shown an increased expression of estrogen and progesterone hormones, suggesting the role of hormonal influence on the lesions.

References

1. Griffith, C. E.M., & Baker, J. (Eds.). (2016). Rook's Textbook of Dermatology (9th ed., Vol. 3). Willey Blackwell.

2. Ingber, A. (2008). Obstetric Dermatology: A Practical Guide. Springer.

3. Tyler, K. H. (Ed.). (2020). Cutaneous Disorders of Pregnancy. Springer International Publishing.

4. Tierney E, Kroumpouzos G, Rogers G. Skin tumors. In: Kroumpouzos G, ed. Text Atlas of Obstetric Dermatology. Philadelphia, PA: Lippincott Williams & Wilkins; 2013. p. 141-151.

5. Walker JL, Wang AR, Kroumpouzos G, Weinstock MA. Cutaneous tumors in pregnancy. Clin Dermatol. 2016;34(3):359–67. https://doi.org/10.1016/j.clindermatol.2016.02.008

6. ChanMP, ChanMM, Tahan SR. Melanocytic nevi in pregnancy: histologic features and Ki-67 proliferation index. J Cutan Pathol. 2010;37:843-851.

7. Zampino MR, Corazza M, Costantino D, et al. Are melanocytic nevi influenced by pregnancy? A dermoscopic evaluation. Dermatol Surg. 2006;32:1497-1504.

8. Andersson TM, Johansson AL, Fredriksson I, et al. Cancer during pregnancy and the postpartum period: a population-based study. Cancer. 2015;121:2072-2077.

9. Lens M, Bataille V. Melanoma in relation to reproductive and hormonal factors in women: current review on controversial issues. Cancer Causes Control. 2008;19:437-442.

10. O'Meara AT, Cress R, Xing G, et al. Malignant melanoma in pregnancy. A population-based evaluation. Cancer. 2005;103:1217-1226.

11. Pugi J, Levin M, Gupta M. Supraglottic p16+ squamous cell carcinoma during pregnancy: a case report and review of the literature. J Otolaryngol Head Neck Surg. 2019;48(1):47. https://doi.org/10.1186/s40463-019-0378-z.

12. Murphy J, Berman DR, Edwards SP, Prisciandaro J, Eisbruch A, Ward BB. Squamous cell carcinoma of the tongue during pregnancy: a case report and review of the literature. J Oral Maxillofac Surg. 2016;74(12):2557–66.

    https://doi.org/10.1016/j.joms.2016.06.173.

13. Fisher GH, Bangash SJ, Mones J, et al. Rapid growth of basal cell carcinoma in a multigestational pregnancy. Dermatol Surg. 2006;32: 1418-1420.

14. Yahya H, Sani H. Eruptive neurofibromas in pregnancy. Ann Afr Med. 2020;19(2):150-152. doi:10.4103/aam.aam_37_19

15. Well L, Jaeger A, Kehrer-Sawatzki H, et al. The effect of pregnancy on growth-dynamics of neurofibromas in Neurofibromatosis type 1. PLoS One. 2020;15(4):e0232031. Published 2020 Apr 28. doi:10.1371/journal.pone.0232031

16. Kuppuswami N, Sivarajan KM, Hussein L, et al. Merkel cell tumor in pregnancy. A case report. J ReprodMed. 1991;36:613-615.

17. Parlette LE, Smith CK, Germain LM, et al. Accelerated growth of dermatofibrosarcoma protuberans during pregnancy. J Am Acad Dermatol. 1999;41:778-783.

18. Brunet-Possenti F, Pages C, Rouzier R, et al. Kaposi's sarcoma and pregnancy: case report and literature review. Dermatology. 2013;226:311-314.

19. Amitay-Layish I, DavidM, Kafri B, et al. Early-stage mycosis fungoides, parapsoriasis en plaque, and pregnancy. Int J Dermatol. 2007;46: 160-165.

Chapter 18

Mucosal Changes In Pregnancy

Introduction

The mucosal changes in pregnancy can be broadly divided into changes occurring in the oral cavity and the genital mucosa. Similar to the changes seen on the skin the mucosal changes can also be physiological or pathological.

The two major mucosal sites which are associated with physiological and pathological changes during pregnancy include the oral mucosa and the genital mucosa. We shall discuss both the physiological and pathological changes occurring in the oral and genital mucosa one by one in this chapter.

Figure 6.

MUCOSAL CHANGES IN PREGNANCY

- Changes in Oral Mucosa
  - Physiological
    - Gingival Hyperemia & Edema.

- Pathological
  - Pyogenic Granuloma
  - Aphthous Ulcers
  - Behcet's Disease
  - Pemphigus Vulgaris
  - Generalised Pustular Psoriasis of Pregnancy
  - Miscellaneous Dermatoses
  - Cheilitis

Changes in Genital Mucosa

Changes in the Oral Mucosa

The changes which are seen in the oral mucosa during pregnancy are predominantly a result of hormonal changes which happen during pregnancy. The increased levels of estrogen and progesterone hormones during pregnancy are believed to contribute to the increased vascularity and decreased cell mediated immunity affecting the oral mucosa. This leads to increased gingival hyperemia and edema and an increased tendency of gingival inflammation and gingival infections. The salivary gland secretions also undergo change in pH and composition during pregnancy. Overall the salivary gland secretion becomes more acidic during pregnancy due to decrease in sodium concentration of saliva. This is often associated with an increased protein concentration. The saliva during pregnancy contains higher levels of estrogen which is believed to increase the proliferation of epithelial cells in the oral mucosa. These changes in the characteristics of saliva contribute to favorable conditions for bacterial superinfections during pregnancy and an increased incidence of dental caries. Changes in the periodontal tissue in the form of gingival hyperemia and erythema, periodontal inflammation and increased tendency of gingival bleeding, increased tooth mobility and higher tendency of dental infections is also seen. The changes in oral mucosa during pregnancy can be broadly classified into physiological and pathological.

Physiological changes in oral mucosa

Gingival hyperemia and edema.

It is seen in more than two thirds of pregnant females. It is also known as *pregnancy gingivitis* and is characterized by edema and hyperplasia of the gingival mucosa. It is benign in most of the cases and the patients usually remain asymptomatic. Some severe cases may present with bleeding and periodontitis. Most of the patients presenting with symptomatic bleeding or pain often have pre-existing gingival inflammation and infection which is exacerbated due to the effect of pregnancy.

Maintenance of good oral hygiene during pregnancy as well as dental care to address pre existing oral conditions can help to improve oral manifestations seen during pregnancy. Conservative dental procedures including scaling are considered safe during pregnancy. In case active dental treatment is required it is advocated to be conducted in the second trimester of pregnancy which is considered safer.

Pathological conditions of oral mucosa.

1. Pyogenic Granuloma (PG)

It is also known as *lobular capillary hemangioma or granuloma gravidarum or epulis of pregnancy*. It is a benign tumor affecting the capillaries and fibroblasts. Almost 2% of the pregnant females can present with pyogenic granuloma during pregnancy. Its increased prevalence in pregnancy is attributed to the increased levels of hormones predominantly estrogen and progesterone during pregnancy. Other factors which have been held responsible for causation of pyogenic granuloma in pregnancy include pregnancy gingivitis, periodontal infections and trauma. Some studies have also suggested the role of vascular endothelial growth factor in causation of PG.

Spontaneous resolution after the completion of pregnancy has been reported in some cases which further reinforces the role of pregnancy associated hormonal surge in its causation. Oral cavity is the most commonly affected site during pregnancy.

It usually presents in the form of a single, painless, bright red coloured, vascular and pedunculated lesion which bleeds easily on manipulation. It commonly develops during the 2 to 5 months of gestation.

As mentioned earlier, some cases of pyogenic granuloma in pregnancy report spontaneous resolution after completion of pregnancy and thus require no active intervention. Intervention can be required in cases of non resolution, frequent bleeding, recurrent infection or large PG. Safer surgical options in pregnancy include electro coagulation, curettage and cryotherapy.

2. Aphthous Ulcers (AU)

Aphthous ulcers can appear afresh during pregnancy or may show more frequent episodes. The exact cause of apthosis is not known however it is often believed to be multifactorial. The role of altered immunological and hormonal balance in pregnancy along with extrinsic factors like deficiencies, infections, food, stress and drugs contributes to the causes of ulcers during pregnancy. The most common presentation is simple aphthous ulcers which usually present as self limiting, sometimes recurrent and often painful superficial oral ulcers limited to non keratinized part of oral mucosa. Some patients may present with complex aphthous ulcers which are usually larger, persist for a longer time of more than 10 days and often heal with scarring.

Aphthous ulcers during pregnancy are to be managed conservatively as most of the ulcers are self limiting and benign in nature. Nutritional deficiencies in the form of iron, folic acid, zinc and vitamin B12 deficiency should be screened and appropriately treated. In case of persistent or problematic ulcers topical orabase or gel based preparations of corticosteroids can help decrease the symptoms and improve resolution of these ulcers. In non responsive cases a short course of oral corticosteroids may be given. Other medications like oral dapsone and colchicine are effective in the treatment of aphthous ulcers however they should be reserved for only non responsive and complicated cases of aphthous ulcers considering their risk benefit equation. Thalidomide which is sometimes used in treatment of aphthous ulcers in the non pregnant population is to be strictly avoided in pregnant females as it is a teratogenic drug and pregnancy category X, and is absolutely contraindicated during pregnancy.

3. Bechet's disease (BD)

Bechet's disease is a chronic multisystem inflammatory disease characterized by recurrent mucosal, ocular, neurological and cutaneous manifestations.

It is seen more commonly in females especially during the third and fourth decade of life. The exact etiology of Bechet's disease is not known, however the role of genetic predisposition and association with HLA B51 allele has been reported. The disease can often be triggered by exogenous insults in the form of drugs, infections and concomitant inflammatory disorders in predisposed individuals resulting in multisystem inflammation and vasculitis.

BD in pregnancy often presents as recurrent oral and or genital ulcers. Other systems which are less commonly involved include the ocular, vascular, cutaneous and nervous system.

Oral lesions which are usually the initial presentation of the disease can present in the form of recurrent aphthous ulcers which are often multiple and painful. The disease follows a course of remissions and relapses.

As far as the effect of pregnancy on BD is concerned, pregnancy overall had a variable effect on BD with around half of the patients reporting improvement in the disease during pregnancy whereas around 27% reported worsening and the rest 20% had no change in the severity of disease as per a study. The resolution of symptoms during pregnancy in a large proportion of patients is attributed to increased levels of sex hormones during pregnancy especially estrogen and progesterone.

As far as the effect of BD on pregnancy is concerned, it was found that it does not adversely affect the maternal or fetal outcome during pregnancy.

The treatment of oral manifestations of behcet's disease in pregnancy is similar to that of aphthous ulcers as discussed above.

4. Oral Involvement in Pemphigus Vulgaris (PV)

Pemphigus vulgaris is an autoimmune vesiculobullous disorder affecting the skin and mucosal sites. Oral lesions in PV can present in the form of flaccid bullae and or erosions that heal slowly on treatment but usually without scarring. Oral mucosa is one of the commonly affected sites and sometimes it is the first or only site to be involved in a case of PV.

The oral erosions in PV can cause difficulty in food intake, affecting the nutritional need in pregnant females. Some females may present with desquamative gingivitis and extensive erosions of the oral and genital mucosa which often heal with difficulty and can show peripheral extension.

PV can show worsening during the course of pregnancy and less commonly can present for the first time during pregnancy. The disease exacerbations are seen more commonly during the first and second trimester. Some cases have shown stabilization of the disease or partial improvement during the third trimester of pregnancy. The improvement is attributed to the production of placental steroids during the later half of pregnancy.

Pemphigus vulgaris in pregnancy has been associated with the occurrence of neonatal pemphigus due to trans-placental diffusion of pathogenic autoantibodies. There have also been reports of adverse neonatal outcomes in females suffering from PV during pregnancy.

The condition has been described in detail in chapter 10 of this book.

5. Oral Involvement in Generalized Pustular psoriasis of Pregnancy (GPP)

It is also known as *impetigo herpetiformis*. It is now more commonly believed to be a variant of generalized pustular psoriasis, with pregnancy acting as a triggering factor.

The disease commonly presents with constitutional symptoms like fever, malaise, myalgias etc. along with skin lesions in the form of the erythematous annular and polycyclic plaques with multiple small pustules coalescing to form lakes of pus. The eruption usually favors the intertriginous and flexural areas. Some cases have been associated with hypoparathyroidism and low calcium levels in the blood.

Oral involvement, though less common, has been reported in association with GPP. The most common presentation is the appearance of a **geographic tongue** which presents in the form of a migratory, geographic pattern of papillary atrophy with raised whitish margins presenting commonly on the dorsum and lateral border of the tongue. Geographic tongue is usually asymptomatic and is encountered as an incidental finding in patients of GPP on examination.

Laboratory investigation may reveal raised leukocyte count and erythrocytes sedimentation rate.

GPP has been described in detail in chapter 8 of this book under the heading of generalized pustular psoriasis of pregnancy.

6. Oral Involvement in other Dermatoses

Other diseases which have been reported with oral involvement in pregnant females include **systemic lupus erythematosus** which can uncommonly present with chronic ulcers typically involving the hard palate and can be treated with topical corticosteroids or oral hydroxychloroquine for symptomatic lesions.

Another disease which can present with oral lesions during pregnancy is **Erythema Multiforme (EM)** although its occurrence during pregnancy has been rarely reported.

Pemphigoid Gestationis (PG) is another less common autoimmune vesiculobullous disorder seen specifically in pregnancy especially during the third trimester or postpartum period. It is characterized by an autoantibody mediated damage to the basement membrane presenting in the form of blistering at the level of dermo-epidermal junction. Clinically it presents in the form of tense vesicles and bullae in pregnant females predominantly affecting the skin of trunk and limbs. Mucosa is usually not involved but rarely vesicles and erosions can extend on to the mucosal sites. PG carries risk of adverse fetal outcomes in pregnancy and needs to be adequately diagnosed and treated. The topic of Pemphigoid gestationis has been dealt in detail in the chapter 5 of this book.

7. Cheilitis during pregnancy

Mucosal involvement of lip (cheilitis) during pregnancy can present commonly in the form of angular cheilitis which is commonly seen due to nutritional deficiency of iron and vitamin B12. Angular cheilitis in pregnancy can also be a part of oral candidal infection. Some females can also present with diffuse involvement of lips with or without associated skin involvement in atopic patients which is known as **atopic cheilitis**. It can be treated conservatively with the use of lip moisturizers and low potency topical steroids.

Changes In The Genital Mucosa During Pregnancy

The hormonal and immunological changes which take place during pregnancy also affect the vaginal mucosa. Pregnancy is associated with changes in the vaginal mucosa in the form of increased edema and vascularity. This manifests clinically in the form of increased vaginal hyperemia and edema giving it a bluish tinge in appearance which is known as the **Chadwick sign**. Increased erythema and edema of the cervix manifest in the form of the **Goodell sign** which is analogous to its vaginal counterpart. The vaginal mucosa becomes more thick during pregnancy with the enlargement of vaginal papillae and vaginal rugosities. Vaginal cellular and biochemical changes in the form of increased epithelial cell turnover, increase in glycogen-containing vaginal discharge and decreased vaginal pH manifest in the form of thin homogenous whitish vaginal discharge which is more acidic in nature. This is often associated with enlargement of underlying vaginal smooth muscles and connective tissue structure. These changes are physiological and aim at preparing the birth canal for the event of childbirth.

The increased blood volume and venous pressure during pregnancy can present as vulvar varicosities and anal hemorrhoids. Venous distension in the vestibule and vulva is known as **Jacquemier sign.**

Pathological conditions affecting the vulva

Most of the pathological conditions in pregnancy which affect the genital mucosa include the Vascular pathologies like hemorrhoids and vulvovaginal infections like candidiasis, bacterial vaginosis, trichomonas infection, and viral infections like genital warts, genital herpes simplex etc.

Vascular disorders of vulvar region

Vascular disorders in the form of anal hemorrhoids and varicosities are commonly seen during pregnancy, however they are mostly benign or asymptomatic and often regress postpartum.

Uncommonly, diseases involving the inguinal skin, perianal or perineal skin can extend or communicate with the genital mucosa. Some examples of these disorders include hidradenitis suppurativa and fox fordyce disease. Henceforth in this chapter we shall discuss the infectious conditions affecting the genital mucosa during pregnancy because of their significance in pregnancy and sometimes the need of active treatment.

Infectious diseases affecting the genital mucosa in pregnancy

1. Vulvovaginal Candidiasis (VVC)

It is a fungal infection affecting the vulvovaginal mucosa caused by a yeast known as *Candida*. Candida sp. is a normal commensal in vaginal mucosa in 25% of the females of reproductive age group. Candidiasis is the second most common cause of vulvovaginal infection after bacterial vaginosis. Pregnancy provides a favorable environment for growth of candida sp. due to the immunological and hormonal changes which take place during the course of pregnancy. The change in biochemical characteristics of vaginal secretions during pregnancy as well as altered cellular immune response promotes the growth of Candida during pregnancy. High levels of estrogen hormone during pregnancy resulting in the increased production of glycogen in the vaginal secretions has also been found to promote candidal infection.

Studies have shown that there is an increased tendency of pregnant females to acquire vulvovaginal candidiasis which is often symptomatic and more severe during pregnancy as compared to non pregnant females. The incidence of VVC during pregnancy is maximum during the second and third trimester.

There is evidence of an increased risk of fetal complications associated with genital candidal infections in the pregnant female. The complications include premature rupture of membrane, preterm delivery, chorioamnionitis and congenital candidiasis. Candidal infection rarely acquired by the fetus while in utero can rarely result in **congenital candidiasis**. Factors like early rupture of membrane, the presence of uterine or cervical foreign body or history of vaginal candidiasis can increase the risk of candidal infection in utero. Another similar condition known as neonatal candidiasis which occurs during the early postpartum period can result due to the infection acquired by the neonate during delivery through the birth canal.

Clinical features include complaints like vaginal itching, burning micturition and pain during intercourse. On examination there may be presence of thick curdy white discharge along with excoriations over the vulva and vaginal mucosa. The surrounding perineum and perianal area and groins may also show signs of candidal intertrigo.

A simple bedside test to demonstrate the presence of fungal yeasts of candida can be done by microscopic examination of vaginal discharge using 10% KOH. Confirmation of diagnosis can be done through fungal culture.

Most of the vulvovaginal infections with candida sp. are asymptomatic and do not require treatment. Candidal infection in pregnant females is to be treated only when symptomatic. There are reports of reduction in risk of preterm birth on proper treatment and eradication of candidal infection during pregnancy. The treatment for symptomatic candidal infection in pregnancy is done using topical imidazole cream or gel like clotrimazole, miconazole or with topical nystatin which is applied locally; or with the use of vaginal pessaries so as to prevent systemic drug exposure of oral antifungals during pregnancy. Oral fluconazole and other oral antifungals are best avoided during pregnancy especially during the first trimester as use of higher doses during pregnancy have shown evidence of fetal toxicity and malformations.

2. Bacterial vaginosis

It is the most common type of vulvovaginal infection seen in pregnant females in the United States. It is characterized by an abnormal shift of vaginal flora from normally present lactobacillus predominant to anaerobic bacteria predominant composition. The anaerobic bacteria which predominate in bacterial vaginosis include gardanarela vaginalis, mobiluncus sp. and mycoplasma sp.

Clinical diagnosis is made using **Amsel's criteria** which includes: (a) vaginal pH of more than 4.5; (b) A fishy or ammoniacal smell of vaginal discharge on adding a drop of potassium hydroxide (**Whiff Test**); (c) Presence of clue cells which are vaginal squamous epithelial cells coated on its margins with lactobacilli and WBCs and (d) The presence of a homogenous vaginal discharge.

There have been reports of adverse fetal outcomes associated with bacterial vaginosis during pregnancy in the form of chorioamnionitis, preterm birth and endometritis however the evidence to suggest prevention of these complications with treatment during pregnancy is lacking.

Treatment of bacterial vaginosis during pregnancy can be done using topical preparation of clindamycin 2% cream which is to be applied for 7 nights consecutively. Topical treatment is specially preferred during the first trimester of pregnancy in order to avoid systemic exposure of medications and its side effects. Oral treatment in the form of metronidazole 400 mg thrice daily for 7 days can be given during the second and third trimester of pregnancy. The combination of oral metronidazole and erythromycin has been reported to improve the pregnancy outcome with respect to preterm birth as compared to placebo.

Oral clindamycin tablets given in the dose of 200 mg for 7 days during the second and third trimester have been shown to be safe in pregnancy however it can result in pseudomembranous colitis especially on long term use.

3. Trichomonal vaginitis

It is a vulvovaginal infection caused by a protozoan known as *trichomonas vaginalis*. It is a flagellate, racket shaped/pyriform organism with a characteristic motility. Trichomonas infection is typically seen in sexually active females. It is seen to be associated with low socioeconomic status and with human immunodeficiency virus infection.

Clinically it can remain asymptomatic but more commonly presents as intense itching and burning involving the vulvovaginal region. Other complaints like burning maturation, increased frequency of urination and discomfort during coitus can be associated. Clinical examination can reveal intense erythema affecting the vulva, vagina and cervix known as **strawberry cervix or colpitis macularis**. The discharge is typically foul smelling and yellow green in color and is often seen adhering to the vaginal wall.

A useful bedside test which can be performed using the vaginal discharge diluted with a few drops of saline can show the motile flagellated organism when viewed under a microscope. The organism appears as a tennis racket shaped or ovoid flagellated and motile structure which is larger than this surrounding WBCs. Demonstration of trichomonas is confirmative of trichomonas vaginal infection.

Vulvovaginal infection with trichomonas is associated with adverse pregnancy outcome especially of the fetus in the form of preterm birth, premature rupture of membrane and intrauterine growth retardation. Maternal complications in the form of infertility and abnormalities in the cervix cytology can be seen.

Thus treatment of trichomonas infection becomes important. Treatment is done using oral metronidazole 250 mg thrice daily or 500 mg twice daily for 7 to 10 days during the second or third trimester of pregnancy. Treatment of trichomonas infection has also shown to decrease the incidence of HIV coinfection in sexually active females.

4. Genital warts

It is caused due to infection by a group of viruses known as human papilloma viruses (HPV). It can present in a number of ways clinically ranging from an asymptomatic infection to the presence of genital warts to genital malignancies. HPV infections are characterized clinically by epithelial tissue proliferations which can present as mucocutaneous watts or as invasive tumors. Based on the oncogenic risk HPV viruses are classified as high risk, intermediate risk and low risk. HPV 16, 18, 45 and 56 carry the highest risk of neoplastic transformation followed by type 31, 33, 35, 39, 51, 52, 58 and 66 which are classified as intermediate risk HPV. Type 6 and 11 are the most common HPV types responsible for causation of genital warts. There have been some reports of increased risk of fetal defects due to HPV infections. Other complications which can arise for the fetus due to HPV infection in the mother during pregnancy include the risk of preterm delivery and respiratory papillomatosis of the neonate during delivery.

Clinically genital warts present in the form of pale or gray coloured fleshy papillated or cauliflower shaped, exophytic, sessile or pedunculated growths involving the vulva, vagina or cervix.

As far as the effect of pregnancy on warts is concerned, genital warts during pregnancy may become larger in size and more friable. Very large genital warts in pregnancy, bleeding warts and those obstructing the birth canal can be treated using safer options like electroablation, carbon dioxide laser ablation, cryotherapy and scalpel excision. Flat warts can be treated with chemical cauterization using trichloroacetic acid. Topical treatments in the form of imiquimod, podophyllin, 5-fluorouracil and interferon should be avoided because of their side effects and risk during pregnancy.

Vaginal delivery can be undertaken in routine cases of HPV as cesarean section delivery is not shown to prevent HPV transmission to the neonate during childbirth. However cesarean section delivery is indicated when the genital warts are large enough to obstruct the birth canal or there is risk of profuse bleeding from the genital warts or when vaginal delivery is otherwise contraindicated.

Preventive measures include administration of bivalent, quadrivalent or the new nonavalent HPV vaccine in females of more than 12 years of age. However they are not to be used during pregnancy.

5. Genital herpes

Genital herpes is a viral infection caused by a double stranded DNA virus known as ***Herpes Simplex Virus*** (HSV) 1 and 2. Herpes simplex type 2 virus is predominantly spread through sexual contact in sexually active males and females. However there is an increased prevalence of HSV 1 causing genital infection nowadays accounting for around 50% of the total cases of genital herpes.

The risk factors for acquiring herpes simplex infection of the genitalia include lower socioeconomic status, low level of education, multiple sexual partners and presence of concomitant sexually transmitted diseases.

Primary genital herpes is defined as genital infection by any subtype of herpes simplex virus (HSV 1 or 2) in a person who has not been infected with either HSV 1 or HSV 2 in the past. It has a longer incubation period of up to 2 weeks and primary genital herpes presents with a more noticeable clinical presentation in the form of multiple painful erosions on the genitalia which can spill over to the adjacent areas like groins, peri anal region, buttocks and the cervix. The ulcers are typically shallow with an erythematous rim. The eruption is often associated with constitutional symptoms like fever, body aches and lethargy. The patient may complain of pain, burning micturition, tender lymphadenopathy and urinary retention. There is active viral proliferation in the lesions and viral shedding may continue for up to three weeks after infection. The virus then goes dormant in the local sensory ganglion and can reactivate later to present as an episode of recurrent herpes.

Recurrent genital herpes infection is less severe in presentation with less chances of systemic symptoms and shorter incubation period along with rapid healing of the erosions which typically appear in a localized and grouped configuration. Recurrent genital herpes is more commonly seen with HSV 2 virus.

The risk in terms of maternal morbidity due to an active genital herpes infection in pregnancy is minimal. However herpes simplex infection being a part of the congenital TORCH complex can have implications for the fetus. A primary infection of genital herpes during pregnancy can present with adverse fetal outcomes in the form of congenital manifestations in the fetus, ocular manifestations and neurological involvement in the form of microcephaly, hydrocephalus and intracranial calcification. Maternal infection of herpes simplex virus around the time of childbirth can lead to development of neonatal herpes.

Asymptomatic shedding of herpes simplex virus can persist in some cases despite the absence of clinical disease. In utero infection can be acquired by the fetus due to the presence of active genital infection in the mother during pregnancy or as a result of asymptomatic viral shedding. The highest risk of transmitting infection to the fetus is in cases of primary genital herpes occurring during the course of pregnancy. Most of such cases are asymptomatic primary episodes and account for around two-thirds of fetal infections.

The fetal prognosis is fairly good when neonates have localized infection of the skin, eyes or mouth due to intrauterine transmission and receive timely intravenous acyclovir therapy at birth. In neonates with disseminated and severe herpes infection with evidence of systemic involvement like liver dysfunction, respiratory or CNS involvement the prognosis is bad. Most of these do not survive and a minority of those who survive suffer from long term deficits.

A pregnant woman who presents with doubtful lesions of genital herpes should be taken up for viral culture for confirmation if the facilities are available. In case the history suggestive of herpes virus infection of the genitalia is present in the absence of any clinical lesions, serological tests in the form of ELISA or immunofluorescence can be taken up. Serological tests however cannot differentiate between HSV type 1 and type 2 infection. Polymerase chain reaction (PCR) detecting herpes simplex virus DNA from the genital swabs or genital erosions is the most sensitive test to detect genital herpes.

Treatment of primary genital herpes includes use of oral acyclovir for the mother in doses of 200 mg 5 times a day or 400 mg thrice daily for 7 to 10 days. In case of recurrent herpes infection of the genitalia, acyclovir in a dose of 400 mg thrice a day for 5 days is sufficient. Acyclovir is a category B drug with a good record of safety in pregnancy. It is shown to decrease the transmission and viral shedding as well as promotes the healing of genital lesions. In females presenting with recurrent episodes of genital herpes during pregnancy, suppressive therapy using acyclovir in doses of 400 mg thrice daily starting from 36 weeks of gestation until delivery can be started. Cesarean section delivery is indicated in females who have active lesions of genital herpes during the time of delivery so as to avoid intrapartum transmission from the mother to the neonate.

6. Molluscum contagiosum

It is a viral infection caused by poxvirus which presents in the form of asymptomatic skin coloured to pearly white umbilicated papules in the genital area of pregnant females. There are chances of transmission of these lesions to the neonate during the time of delivery as a result of skin to skin contact and through fomites. Safe treatment options during pregnancy include curettage, chemical cauterization with trichloroacetic acid and cryotherapy.

References

1. Ingber, A. (2008). Obstetric Dermatology: A Practical Guide. Springer.

2. Tyler, K. H. (Ed.). (2020). Cutaneous Disorders of Pregnancy. Springer International Publishing.

3. Barak S, Oettinger-Barak O, Oettinger M, et al. Common oral manifestations during pregnancy: a review. Obstet Gynecol Surv 2003;58:624- 8.

4. Ramos-E-Silva M, Martins NR, Kroumpouzos G. Oral and vulvovaginal changes in pregnancy. Clin Dermatol. 2016 May-Jun;34(3):353-8. doi: 10.1016/j.clindermatol.2016.02.007. Epub 2016 Mar 2. PMID: 27265073.

5. Torgerson RR, Marnach ML, Bruce AJ, Rogers RS 3rd. Oral and vulvar changes in pregnancy. Clin Dermatol. 2006 Mar-Apr;24(2):122-32. doi: 10.1016/j.clindermatol.2005.10.004. PMID: 16487887.

6. Kondo RN, Araújo FM, Pereira AM, Lopes VC, Martins LM. Pustular psoriasis of pregnancy (impetigo herpetiformis)--case report. An Bras Dermatol. 2013;88(6 Suppl 1):186-189. doi:10.1590/abd1806-4841.20132134

7. Muhammad JK, Lewis MA, Crean SJ. Oral pemphigus vulgaris occurring during pregnancy. J Oral Pathol Med. 2002 Feb;31(2):121-4. doi: 10.1046/j.0904-2512.2001.00000.x. PMID: 11896835.

8. Martineau M, Haskard DO, Nelson-Piercy C. Behçet's syndrome in pregnancy. Obstet Med. 2010;3(1):2-7. doi:10.1258/om.2009.090033

9. Annan B, Nuamah K. Oral pathologies seen in pregnant and non-pregnant women. Ghana Med J. 2005;39(1):24-27. doi:10.4314/gmj.v39i1.35977

10. Straface G, Selmin A, Zanardo V, De Santis M, Ercoli A, Scambia G. Herpes simplex virus infection in pregnancy. Infect Dis Obstet Gynecol. 2012;2012:385697.

    doi:10.1155/2012/385697

11. Sugai S, Nishijima K, Enomoto T. Management of Condyloma Acuminata in Pregnancy: A Review. Sex Transm Dis. 2021;48(6):403-409. doi:10.1097/OLQ.0000000000001322

Index

A

Acne vulgaris in pregnancy 125

Acrodermatitis enteropathica (AE) 146

Allergic contact dermatitis, 63

Amsel's criteria 104

Anetoderma 153, 154

Antiphospholipid antibody syndrome (APLAS) 84

Aphthous ulcers (AU) 180

Apocrine gland diseases in pregnancy 135

Atopic dermatitis 50, 60, 61, 75

Autoimmune progesterone dermatitis in pregnancy 159

B

Bacterial vaginosis 19, 104, 121, 190

Bechet's disease (BD) 181

C

Carpal tunnel syndrome 21

Changes in melanocytic lesions in pregnancy 167

Changes in the genital mucosa during pregnancy 186

Changes in the hair during pregnancy 14

Changes in the nails during pregnancy 16

Changes in the oral mucosa 176

Cheilitis during pregnancy 186

Chicken pox in a neonate 109

Congenital varicella syndrome 108

Connective tissue changes 9, 13

D

Dermatomyositis and pregnancy 90

Dermatomyositis (DM) 89

E

Eccrine glands diseases in pregnancy 137

Edema of pregnancy 19

Effect of pregnancy on psoriasis 65

Effect of psoriasis on pregnancy 65

Ehler danlos syndrome (EDS) 155

Ehler danlos syndrome and pregnancy 155

Erythema nodosum (EN) 73

F

Fox fordyce disease (FFD) 135, 136

G

Generalized pustular psoriasis of pregnancy (GPP) 67

Genital herpes 112, 184

Genital warts 19, 110, 182

Genital warts in pregnancy 110

Gingival erythema and hyperemia 17

Gingival hyperemia and edema 177

Glandular changes in pregnancy 21

H

Hematological and hemodynamic changes in pregnancy 21

Herpes simplex infection in pregnancy 112

Herpes zoster and chickenpox infection in pregnancy 106

Herpes zoster infection in pregnancy 106

Hidradenitis suppurativa (HS) 135

Hirsutism 9, 15

Human immunodeficiency virus (HIV) infection in pregnancy 115

Hyperhidrosis 137

I

Infantile herpes zoster 108

Infectious diseases affecting the genital mucosa in pregnancy 188

L

Leprosy in pregnancy 120

Linear igm dermatoses (LID) of pregnancy 163

Lupus erythematosus (LE) 79

M

Malignant melanoma (MM) 167

Malignant melanoma in pregnancy 167, 173

Miliaria 137

Molluscum contagiosum 187

Mucosal changes in pregnancy 175

N

Neonatal lupus erythematosus 83

Neurofibromatosis 169, 173

Neurovascular changes in pregnancy 17

Non-melanoma skin cancers (NMSCS) 166

O

Oral involvement in generalized pustular psoriasis of pregnancy (GPP) 183

Oral involvement in other dermatoses 185

Oral involvement in pemphigus vulgaris (PV) 182

Other tumorous growths in pregnancy 169

P

Palmar erythema 18

Pathological conditions affecting the vulva 187

Pathological conditions of oral mucosa 179

Pemphigus and pregnancy 97, 100, 101

Pemphigus foliaceus (PF) 98

Pemphigus foliaceus and pregnancy 98

Pemphigus vulgaris (PV) 95

Physiological changes in oral mucosa 177

Physiological changes in pregnancy 9

Pityriasis rosea in pregnancy 114, 123

Porphyria cutanea tarda (PCT) 141

Postpartum telogen effluvium 9, 14

Pregnancy induced pigmentation 10

Pregnancy specific dermatoses 29

Pseudoxanthoma elasticum (PXE) 151

Psoriasis 64, 65

Pxe and pregnancy 152

Pyogenic granuloma (PG) 179

Pyogenic granuloma of pregnancy 17

R

Rosacea in pregnancy 129

S

Scabies in pregnancy 119

Skin diseases in pregnancy 1, 5

Skin tags 14

Spider angioma 18

Striae gravidarum 13

Syphilis in pregnancy 118, 124

Systemic sclerosis (SS) 85

Systemic sclerosis and pregnancy 86

T

Trichomonal Vaginitis 19, 105, 181

U

Urticaria 71, 72, 77

V

Varicella/chickenpox in pregnancy 107

Vascular disorders of vulvar region 187

Venous varicosities 19

Vulvovaginal candidiasis 103, 121

Vulvovaginal candidiasis (VVC) 188

www.ingramcontent.com/pod-product-compliance
Ingram Content Group UK Ltd.
Pitfield, Milton Keynes, MK11 3LW, UK
UKHW020244240426
12048UKWH00026B/1607